DASH DIET COOKBOOK FOR BEGINNERS 2024

Quick and Easy-to-Follow Delicious Low Sodium Recipes for Healthy Heart, Weight Loss and Overcome Hypertension

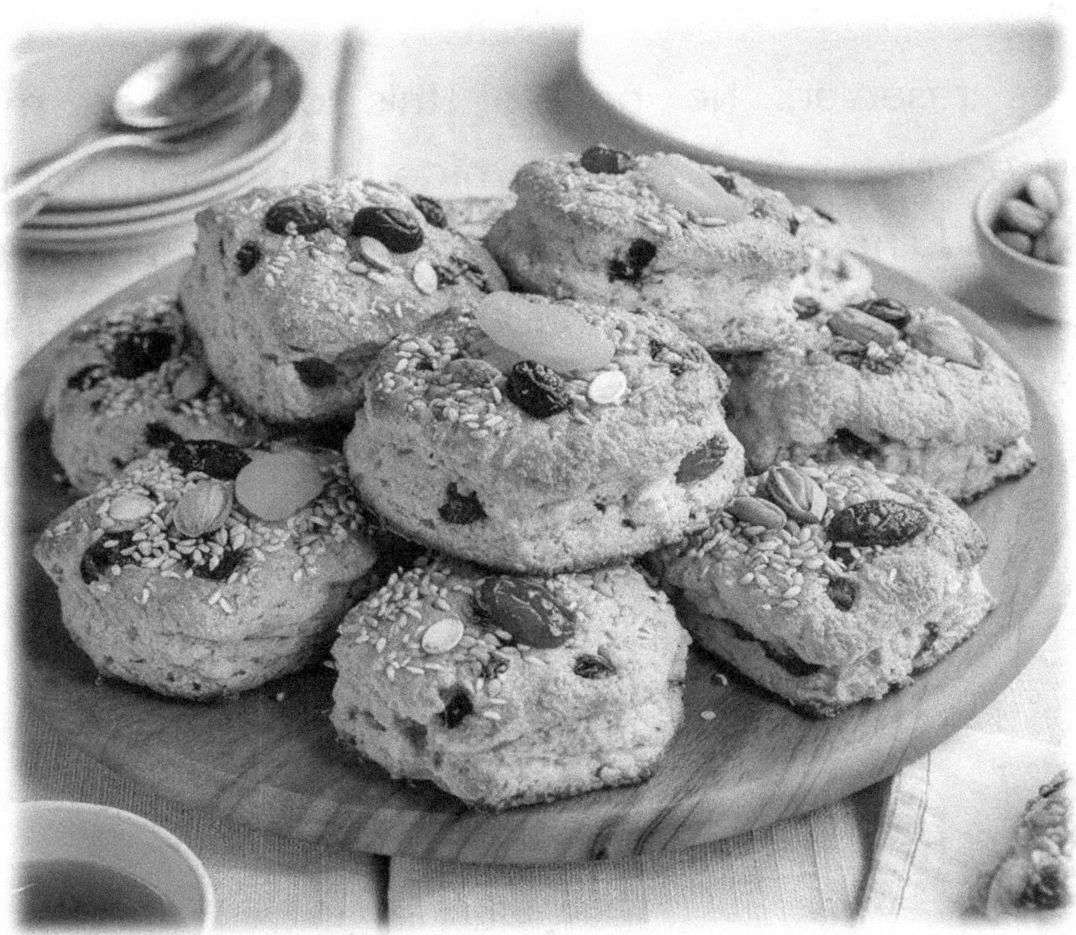

Cynthia Ashcroft

Copyright © 2024 by Cynthia Ashcroft

Thank You for Coming Onboard!

I am very happy to go with you on this new life-changing Dash Diet journey! This book is made to inform you, guide you, and inspire you every step and bite of the way. It has helpful tricks, insights, and practical recipes.

The recipes include breakfast, lunch, dinner, sides, dessert and snack treats. But your journey does not end when you get to the final page of this book.

At the end of this cookbook (paper version), you will find a special **30 day meal plan and free 4 week meal planner journal** to support your Dash diet journey.

Use these resources to find your favorite dishes and plan your Dash diet experience based on the foods you like and what you need.

I'm over the moon that you will get to experience all the delicious recipes I have poured my heart into creating.

Get ready for a flavor adventure! Cheers to healthy and tasty meals ahead!

About Me

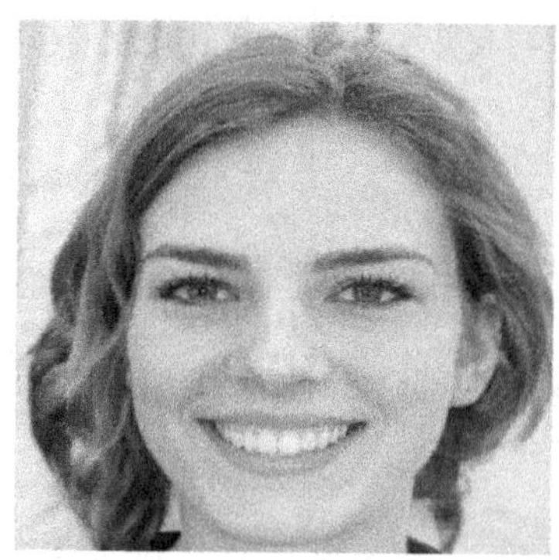

Cynthia Ashcroft is a great cook and food expert who loves everything about eating good foods and living a nice life. She knows a lot about making tasty meals and how the foods we eat make our bodies feel.

Cynthia liked cooking since she was very young. She decided to learn all about it by going to cooking schools and working with experienced chefs.

But she didn't stop there. She also studied a lot about what foods do for our bodies. She wanted to understand how foods can make us feel better and stay healthy.

Cynthia thinks cooking and eating right are very important. She makes foods that not only taste good but are also good for you. She believes you don't have to give up yummy food to eat healthy. You just need to know what is in your foods and choose things that are good for your body.

Cynthia shares her cooking tricks and health tips in books and stories. She helps people eat better without getting tired of their meals.

In her life, Cynthia loves being active and trying new recipes with her husband. They like going on fun trips outside and living the healthy lifestyle Cynthia talks about.

She shows that eating right and staying active can be fun and make you feel good.

Cynthia wants to help you see that healthy food can be enjoyed without feeling bad about breaking diet rules.

TABLE OF CONTENT

INTRODUCTION

A Testament to Transformation

Working towards improved health can be daunting, but it can also be incredibly rewarding. Whitney was introduced to the DASH Diet at a critical point in her life. She struggled with high blood pressure at age 43, coupled with a strong family history of heart disease. She was determined to make a change but the transformation would not happen overnight. Whitney took her time learning about the different diets out there. She finally chose to stick with the Dash diet. Adapting to this new way of eating was daunting at first, but gradually she overcame all setbacks thanks to the guidance of this cookbook. The positive changes were evident in Whitney's health metrics, energy levels, and overall vitality. This cookbook is a culmination of my experiences and knowledge to guide you through similar positive changes Whitney enjoyed easily and confidently.

Key Principles of the DASH Diet

The Dietary Approaches to Stop Hypertension (DASH) Diet is celebrated for its effectiveness in lowering blood pressure and improving overall cardiovascular health. At its core, the DASH Diet emphasizes:

✓ Rich intakes of fruits, vegetables, and whole grains.

✓ Incorporation of dairy products, fish, poultry, beans, seeds, and nuts.

✓ Limited amounts of fats, red meats, sweets, and sugary beverages.

✓ This dietary pattern not only supports heart health but also fosters overall well-being, making it relevant in today's health-conscious society.

This approach not only helps in reducing blood pressure but also supports overall health by promoting weight management, reducing cancer risk, and stabilizing blood sugar levels.

Unique Approach of This Cookbook

This cookbook is crafted to make the DASH Diet approachable and enjoyable. Each recipe is designed to deliver maximum flavor with minimum fuss, helping you to integrate heart-healthy meals into your daily routine effortlessly. The recipes are diverse, catering to various tastes and dietary needs, ensuring that everyone can find something to enjoy. Furthermore, the cookbook simplifies the science behind the diet, providing practical tips on how to make each meal both nutritious and delicious. By focusing on flavor and ease, this cookbook aims to make healthy eating a pleasure, not a chore.

UNDERSTANDING THE DASH DIET

Origins and Evolution of the Dash Diet

The journey of the DASH Diet began in the early 1990s when researchers were searching for ways to naturally reduce high blood pressure without the use of medications. Initiated through trials sponsored by the National Institutes of Health, the DASH Diet quickly demonstrated its potential. These studies were pivotal, revealing that dietary adjustments could significantly impact blood pressure levels. Over the years, the DASH Diet has evolved from a clinical recommendation to a widely accepted and celebrated eating plan, recognized for its broad range of health benefits and its adaptability to different lifestyles and preferences.

Main Components of the Diet

Understanding the components of the DASH Diet is crucial for incorporating its principles into daily life. Here's a detailed look at each group:

➢ **Fruits and Vegetables:** These provide essential vitamins, minerals, and fibers that help reduce blood pressure and support overall health. A variety of colors and types ensures a broad spectrum of nutrients.

➢ **Whole Grains:** These are vital for heart health and maintaining steady energy levels throughout the day. Whole grains are richer in fiber and nutrients compared to refined grains, which helps in managing cholesterol and blood sugar levels.

➢ **Lean Proteins:** This component focuses on meats with lower fat content and plant-based proteins that are beneficial for heart health. Lean proteins help in building and repairing body tissues without adding excessive saturated fats.

➢ **Dairy:** The inclusion of low-fat or fat-free dairy products provides calcium, vitamin D, and protein, crucial for bone health and blood pressure regulation.

➢ **Nuts, Seeds, and Legumes:** These are included a few times a week to provide additional proteins, healthy fats, and fibers, which contribute to satiety and metabolic health.

➢ **Fats and Oils:** The diet emphasizes healthy fats, such as those found in olive oil, avocados, and certain fish, which can have a positive effect on heart health.

Portion Sizes and Daily Recommendations

The DASH Diet also specifies portion sizes and daily intake recommendations to maximize health benefits:

✓ Fruits and Vegetables: 4 to 5 servings each per day.

✓ Whole Grains: 6 to 8 servings per day.

✓ Lean Proteins: Depending on individual needs, 2 to 6 servings per day.

✓ Dairy: 2 to 3 servings per day.

✓ Nuts, Seeds, and Legumes: 4 to 5 servings per week.

✓ Fats and Oils: 2 to 3 servings per day.

Scientific Evidence Supporting Health Benefits

Extensive research has validated the DASH Diet's effectiveness in promoting health and preventing disease. Key findings include its ability to quickly lower blood pressure and its long-term benefits for heart health. Further studies have linked the DASH Diet to reduced risks of cancer, stroke, and diabetes, underscoring its role in overall health maintenance and disease prevention. The comprehensive nature of the diet, with its focus on nutrient-rich and balanced foods, supports not just specific health issues but also contributes to long-term wellness.

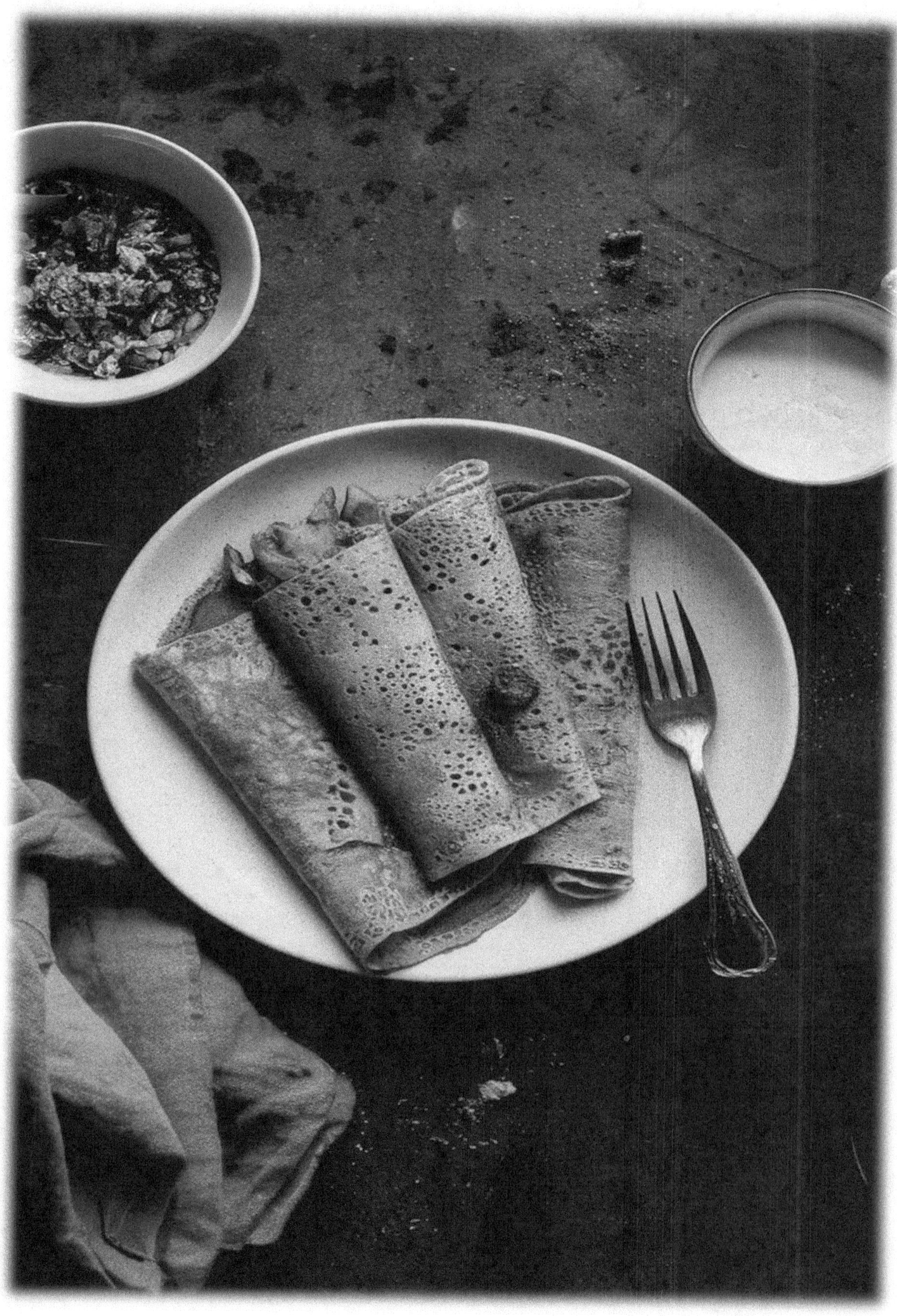

SETTING UP YOUR DASH DIET KITCHEN

Organizing and Stocking a Dash Diet-Friendly Pantry

Creating an environment conducive to healthy eating is crucial for success on the DASH Diet. The pantry is often the starting point for meal preparation, so having it aligned with your dietary goals is essential.

Here are detailed steps to optimize your pantry:

✓ Remove items that are high in sodium, saturated fats, and added sugars. These include processed snacks, canned soups with high sodium content, and sugary cereals.

✓ Fill your pantry with whole grains like barley, bulgur, and oatmeal; legumes such as black beans, kidney beans, and lentils; and various seeds like flaxseeds and chia seeds for added fiber and omega-3 fatty acids.

✓ Build a robust collection of seasonings to enhance flavors without relying on salt. Consider growing a small herb garden in your kitchen for fresh picks like cilantro, parsley, and mint.

✓ Choose heart-healthy options like low-sodium vegetable broths, tomato products without added salts or sugars, and canned fish packed in water.

Essential Kitchen Tools and Gadgets

Equipping your kitchen with the right tools can significantly enhance your cooking experience and help maintain your adherence to the DASH Diet:

➢ **Pressure Cooker or Slow Cooker:** These are excellent for making stews, soups, and beans without added fat and with minimal nutrient loss.

➢ **Quality Non-Stick Cookware:** Reduces the need for cooking oils. Look for PTFE-free and PFOA-free options.

➢ **Salad Spinner:** Makes washing and preparing leafy greens and herbs easy, encouraging you to include more in your diet.

➢ **Digital Food Scale:** Helps with precise portion control, an important aspect of managing your dietary intake according to DASH guidelines.

Strategies for Meal Planning and Grocery Shopping

Effective meal planning and grocery shopping are key components in maintaining the DASH Diet:

➢ Consider theme nights like "Meatless Monday" or "Fish Friday" to add variety and make meal planning easier.

➢ Focus on buying fruits and vegetables that are in season for the best flavor and Nutrition Facts at a lower cost.

➢ Apps and tools can help you track what you eat, plan meals, and even generate shopping lists based on your meal plans.

➢ Participate in local farmer's markets or join a community-supported agriculture (CSA) box to get fresh, seasonal produce directly from farmers.

Building a DASH-Friendly Fridge and Freezer

Beyond the pantry, the refrigerator and freezer also play important roles in a DASH-friendly kitchen. Keep fruits and vegetables at eye level in clear containers to encourage healthier snack choices. Stock frozen vegetables and fruits (without added sugars or sauces), lean protein sources like fish and chicken breast, and whole-grain products like brown rice and whole wheat bread for convenience without compromising on health.

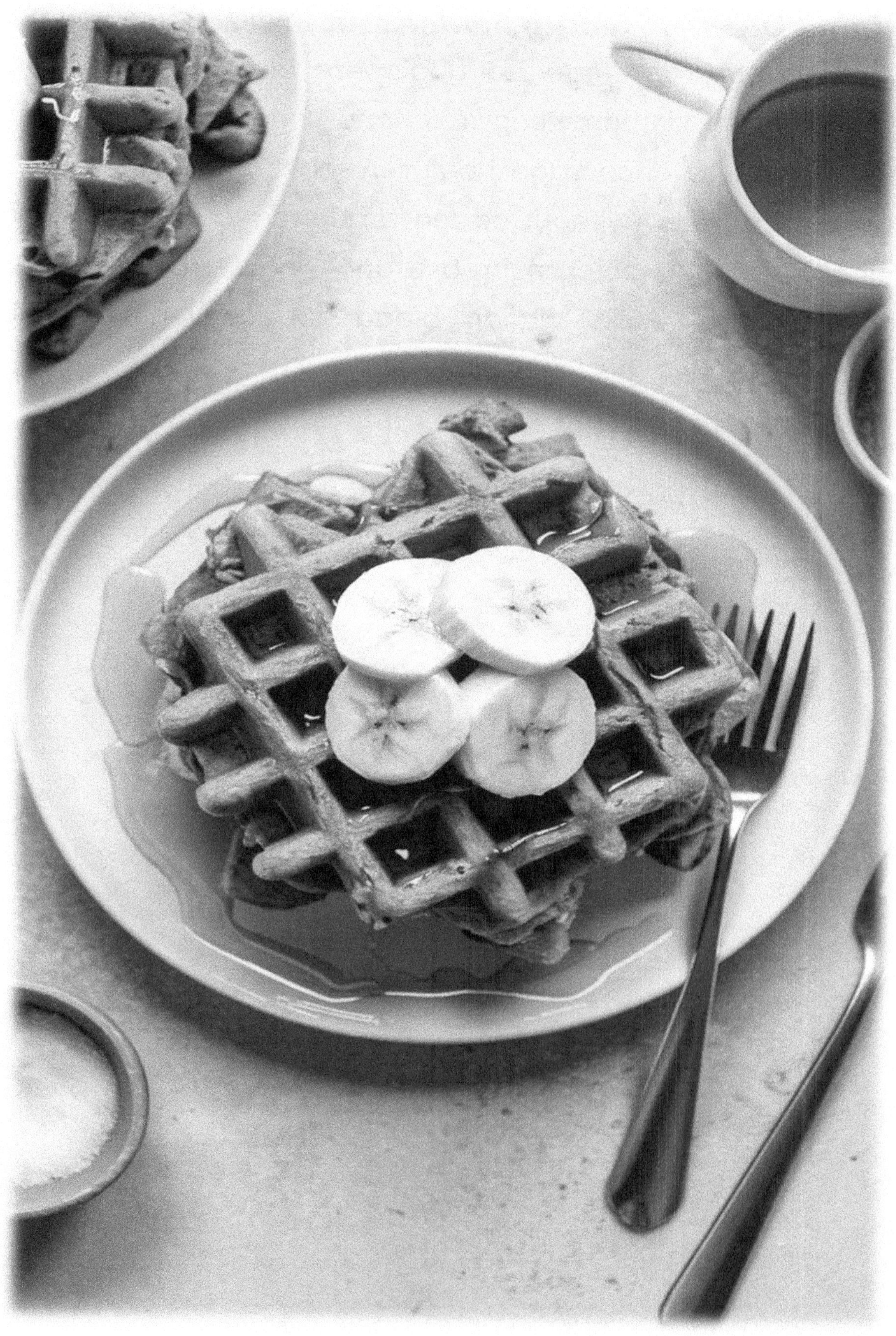

DELIGHTFUL BREAKFAST RECIPES

Peanut Butter Overnight Oats

Serves: 2   **Prep & Cook Time:** 6hours 5mins

Ingredients:

For Oats

- 1 cup unsweetened plain almond milk
- 1.5 Tbsp chia seeds
- 4 Tbsp of natural salted peanut butter or almond butter
- 2 Tbsp maple syrup
- 1 cup gluten-free rolled oats (rolled oats are best)

Optional Toppings

- Sliced bananas, strawberries, or raspberries

Let's Get Cooking:

1. Combine almond milk, chia seeds, peanut butter, and maple syrup (or another sweetener) in a mason jar or a small bowl with a lid. Stir the mixture with a spoon. The peanut butter doesn't need to be fully blended with the almond milk.

2. Add oats and stir a few more times. Then, use a spoon to press down and make sure that all the oats are well covered by the almond milk.

3. Securely cover with a lid or seal and place in the refrigerator overnight, or for at least 6 hours, to allow the oat soak.

4. The next day, open and enjoy as is or choose a topping from options above to garnish.

Nutrition Facts: Calories: 452; Carbs: 51.7g; Protein: 14.6g; Fat: 22.8g

Muesli Scones

Serves: 16 scones   **Prep & Cook Time:** 25mins

Ingredients:

- 2 cups blanched almond flour
- ½ teaspoon celtic sea salt
- ½ teaspoon baking soda
- ¼ cup dried cranberries
- ¼ cup dried apricots (cut into ¼-inch pieces)
- ¼ cup sunflower seeds
- ¼ cup raw sesame seeds
- ¼ cup pistachios, coarsely chopped
- 1 big egg
- 2 tablespoons agave nectar or honey

Let's Get Cooking:

1. Mix almond flour, salt, and baking soda in a big bowl.
2. Stir in dried fruit, seeds and nuts
3. Mix egg and agave in a small bowl
4. Stir wet ingredients into dry
5. Use your hands to form dough
6. Shape dough into a square that is about a bit thick. Cut dough into 16 squares
7. Bake at 350ºF on a baking sheet lined with parchment paper for 10-12 minutes. Serve immediately.

Nutrition Facts: Calories: 152; Fat: 10.5g; Carbs: 9.2g; Protein: 4.6g

Healthy Breakfast Cookies

Servings: 24 cookies   **Prep & Cook Time:** 25mins

Ingredients:

- 2 cup creamy peanut butter (or other nut butter)
- 0.5 cup honey
- 2 teaspoon vanilla extract
- 4 medium ripe bananas, mashed
- 1 teaspoon salt
- 2 teaspoon ground cinnamon
- 4.5 cups quick oats
- 1 cup dried cranberries or raisins
- 1 cup chopped nuts, such as almonds, walnuts or pistachios

Let's Get Cooking:

1) Preheat the oven to 325°F, then line your baking sheet it with parchment paper or a silicone mat.

2) Mix the peanut butter, honey, vanilla extract, mashed bananas, salt, and cinnamon together in a bowl or mixer. Add the oats, dried cranberries, and nuts until they are well-mixed.

3) Use a 1/4 cup measure to scoop mounds of the cookie dough onto the baking sheet, gently flattening each one.

4) Bake the cookies for 14 to 16 minutes until they are golden brown and soft. After removing them from the oven, let them cool on the baking sheet for 5 minutes before transferring to a cooling rack to cool completely.

Nutrition Facts: Calories: 276; Carbs: 31g; Protein: 9g; Fat: 15g

Mushroom Spinach Omelet

Servings: 2   **Prep & Cook Time:** 18mins

Ingredients:

- 2 tablespoons olive oil
- 1/2 cup slice of red onion
- 3 cup fresh spinach
- 10 baby bella mushrooms, sliced
- 2 oz goat cheese
- Cooking Spray
- 2 whole egg
- 4 egg whites
- Green onions, diced (for optional garnish)

Let's Get Cooking:

1. Heat up your pan to medium-high heat. Add olive oil and red onions to the pan. Sauté the onions for two to three minutes.
2. Add sliced mushrooms to the pan, and sauté until the mushrooms are slightly browned—approx. 4-5 minutes.
3. Next, add spinach to the pan. Sauté the spinach until it wilts: that should take about 2mins. Season with salt and pepper. Set aside.
4. Heat another pan (or same pan) to medium heat. Spray with cooking spray.
5. Combine one whole egg with two egg whites in a small bowl. Whisk to mix.
6. Add the egg mixture to the pan. Let the mixture sit for one minute. Carefully use a spatula to loosen the edges of the egg from the pan.

7. Raise the pan slightly and tilt it, rotating in a circular motion to allow the uncooked eggs in the center to flow toward the edges you've just cleared.

8. Add the mushroom-spinach mixture to one side of the omelet and top with crumbled goat cheese. Use your spatula to carefully fold the omelet over the side filled with mushrooms and spinach. Allow it to cook for another 30 seconds.

9. Transfer the omelet onto a plate. Top with green onions

Nutrition Facts: Calories: 412; Fat: 29g; Carbs: 18g; Protein: 25g

Blueberry Banana Spelt Muffins

Servings: 12 large muffins   **Prep & Cook time:** 45mins

Ingredients:

- 2 medium ripe bananas (mashed)
- 3/4 cup plus 2 tablespoons of unsweetened almond milk
- 1 teaspoon apple cider vinegar
- 1/4 cup (60 mL) pure maple syrup
- 1 teaspoon pure vanilla extract
- 1/4 cup coconut oil (melted)
- 2 cups (280 g) white spelt flour
- 4 to 6 tablespoons coconut sugar
- 2 teaspoons baking powder
- 1 1/2 teaspoons cinnamon
- 1/2 teaspoon fine-grain sea salt
- 1/2 teaspoon baking soda
- 1/2 cup of walnut halves, chopped (optional)
- 1 1/4 cups frozen or fresh blueberries

Let's Get Cooking:

1. Preheat oven to 350°F (180°C) and grease a muffin tin.
2. Mash the bananas in a bowl and measure out 3/4 cup . Any excess mashed banana can be frozen for use in a smoothie.
3. Combine the mashed banana, milk, vinegar, maple syrup, and vanilla in a medium bowl. No need to stir it yet.
4. Gently melt the coconut oil in a small saucepan over low heat. Set aside.

5. Mix the dry ingredients (flour, sugar, baking powder, cinnamon, salt, and baking soda) in a large bowl.

6. Stir coconut oil into the wet mixture. Combine the wet ingredients with the dry ones, stirring until they are just mixed. Be careful not to over mix, as spelled flour is quite delicate.

7. Carefully fold the walnuts and then the blueberries, taking care not to over mix to avoid making the muffins too dense.

8. Spoon 1/4 cup of batter into each muffin tin, filling each tin about 3/4 full. They will be almost full, but this is normal. I enjoy pressing a few additional blueberries on top before baking to enhance their appearance.

9. Bake at 350°F (180°C) for 23 to 27 minutes, or until a toothpick inserted into the center comes out clean. I baked them for 25 minutes.

10. Cool in pan for 5 to 8 minutes and then transfer muffins to a cooling rack and cool for another 15 minutes.

Note: If you are using ripe bananas, 4 tablespoons of sugar is enough to maintain sweetness. However, if the bananas are not overripe, you may need to use up to 6 tablespoons. When using frozen blueberries, it's important to keep them in the freezer and not thaw them until you're ready to fold them into the batter. This helps prevent bleeding.

Nutrition Facts: Calories: 180 | Fat: 5g | Carbohydrate: 31g | Protein: 4g

5 Ingredient Buckwheat Crepes

Servings: 24 crepes   **Prep & Cook Time:** 25mins

Ingredients:

For Crepes

- 2 cup un-toasted (raw) buckwheat flour (not kasha or Bob's Red Mill)
- 1.5 Tbsp flaxseed meal
- 3.5 cups light (canned) coconut milk
- 2 pinch sea salt
- 2 Tbsp avocado or coconut oil
- 1 tsp ground cinnamon (optional)
- Sweetener (optional)

For Fillings (your choice)

- Compote
- Nut Butter
- Coconut Whipped Cream
- Granola
- Cinnamon Baked Apples

Let's Get Cooking:

1. Add buckwheat flour, flaxseed meal, light coconut milk, salt, avocado oil, cinnamon, and sweetener of choice to a blender or mixing bowl.

2. Blend the ingredients in a blender or whisk them in a mixing bowl to combine. The batter should be pourable but not too liquid. Should the mixture be too thin, incorporate a little more buckwheat flour. If it's too thick, dilute it with additional dairy-free milk.

3. Heat a nonstick pan over medium heat. Once the pan is hot, add a small amount of oil and swirl to coat evenly. Wait until the oil is

sufficiently heated – it should sizzle and evaporate instantly when you sprinkle a few drops of water onto it.

4. Add 1/4 cup (60 ml) batter. Cook until the top is bubbly and the edges are dry, similar to when preparing pancakes. Then carefully flip and cook for 2-3 minutes more on the other side. Reduce the heat if the food is cooking too fast.

5. Repeat until all crepes are prepared. I found that adding more oil wasn't necessary after the first crepe. To keep them warm, place the crepes between layers of parchment paper or cover them on a plate with a towel.

6. Enjoy with a touch of vegan butter, nut butter, maple syrup, compote, or your choice of fillings! I favor vegan butter, berries, maple syrup, and bananas. However, they would also taste great with coconut whipped cream, cinnamon-baked apples, and fresh fruit such as berries bananas, or granola.

Notes: It's best to enjoy it fresh; however, you can keep the leftovers in a sealed container in the refrigerator for up to three days. For freezing, place layers of parchment paper between the items to avoid sticking, and then freeze. Afterward, transfer them to a freezer-safe container where they can be stored for up to one month. When reheating, warm them in an oven set to 350°f (176° Celsius) or microwave until they are hot.

Nutrition Facts/Serving: Calories: 71 | Carbs: 8g | Protein: 1g | Fat: 3g

Blueberry Yogurt Multigrain Pancakes

Serves: 12 to 14 pancakes　　　　　　**Prep & Cook Time:** 25mins

Ingredients:

- 2 large eggs
- 1 cup plain, full-fat yogurt
- 2 to 4 tablespoons milk
- 3 tablespoons of butter
- 1/2 teaspoon lemon zest
- 1/2 teaspoon vanilla extract
- 1/2 cup (62 grams) whole wheat flour
- 1/2 cup (68 grams) all-purpose flour
- 1/4 cup of barley or rye flour
- 2 tablespoons sugar
- 2 tablespoons baking powder
- 1/2 teaspoon table salt
- 1 cup blueberries, rinsed and dried

Let's Get Cooking:

1. Melt half of the butter. Take off the heat and mix in the second tablespoon of butter until it's melted. This method ensures the butter remains at a suitable temperature for when you incorporate it into the wet ingredients.

2. In the bottom of a medium to large bowl, whisk together the egg and yogurt. If the yogurt is thin, there's no need to add milk. For regular yogurt, mix in 2 tablespoons of milk. For thick, strained, or Greek-style yogurt, incorporate 3 to 4 tablespoons of milk. Whisk in the melted butter, zest, and vanilla extract. In a separate smaller bowl, mix the

flour, sugar, baking powder, and salt. Combine the dry ingredients with the wet, stirring just until the dry ingredients are dampened, and it's okay if a few lumps remain.

3. Preheat your oven to 200°F and prepare a baking sheet to keep the pancakes warm. Heat your pan or sauté pan to medium heat. A cast-iron pan is ideal for pancakes. Melt a small amount of butter in it and pour a scant 1/4 cup (about 3 tablespoons) of batter into each pancake, ensuring there is space between them. Place a few berries on top of each pancake. Since the batter is quite thick, use a spoon or spatula to gently flatten it, or simply press the berries down to spread the batter out.

4. When the pancakes are dry around the edges and bubbles appear on the surface, usually after 3 to 4 minutes, flip them. Cook for another 3 minutes until they are golden brown underneath. You might hear the blueberries pop and sizzle enticingly in the pan after a minute. If the pancakes are cooking too fast, reduce the heat. As each pancake finishes cooking, place it in a warm oven where they can stay until you're ready to serve.

Nutrition Facts/Serving: Calories: 110 | Protein: 3g | Fat: 4.5g | Carb: 15g

Sweet Potato Oat Waffles

Serves: 2   **Prep & Cook Time:** 10mins

Ingredients:

- Oats Waffles
- 1/2 Cup Sweet Potato (cooked)
- 1 Cup Oats (whole grain oats)
- 1 Cup Almond Milk (original, unsweetened)
- 2 Egg(s) (1 whole and 1 egg white)
- 1/4 tsp Baking Powder
- 1 tbsp Honey
- 1/4 tsp Salt
- 1 tbsp Olive Oil
- Oil Spray (for waffle iron)
- For Serving; Banana (sliced) & Maple Syrup

Let's Get Cooking:

1. Set the waffle iron to preheat. Place all ingredients into the blender jar and blend until completely pureed. For optimal results, allow the batter to rest for 10 minutes.
2. Spray waffle iron with oil. Pour batter 1/3 cup into each waffle mold. Cook 30 seconds more, after waffle iron indicator turns green or for 3-4 minutes per batch.
3. The waffle is ready when the steam stops coming out from the waffle iron.
4. Serve it with maple syrup and freshly chopped bananas.

Nutrition Facts: Calories: 530 | Carbs: 82g | Protein: 15g | Fat: 18g

Sweet Potato and Black Bean Breakfast Burrito

Serves: 6   **Prep & Cook Time:** 25mins

Ingredients:

- 6 (8-inch) whole wheat tortillas
- 3 medium sweet potatoes
- 1 (15 ounces) of canned black beans (rinse and drain it)
- 1/2 teaspoon cumin
- 1/4 teaspoon chili powder
- few dashes of red pepper flakes, if desired
- 6 large eggs
- 1 avocado, diced
- 1/2 cup shredded Mexican or Colby jack cheese
- 1/3 cup red enchilada sauce

Let's Get Cooking:

1. Pierce the potatoes with a fork several times. Place them in the microwave and cook on high for 4-6 minutes, or until they are cooked through. This process may take up to 10 minutes, depending on the thickness of your sweet potatoes. Or, you can roast them in the oven at 375° for 45 minutes or until fork tender.

2. After cooking the sweet potatoes, peel off the skins and transfer the potatoes to a medium-sized bowl—Mash with a fork; set aside.

3. Combine black beans, cumin, chili powder, and red pepper flakes, if desired in a separate large bowl. Stir to combine then set aside.

4. Beat the eggs (or egg whites) together in a separate medium bowl. Coat a pan with nonstick cooking spray and set it over medium-low

heat. Add in eggs and cook. Fold every few minutes to get fluffy eggs. Once cooked, remove from heat.

5. For the burrito, ensure the tortillas are slightly warm to facilitate easier rolling. Warm them in the microwave for 10-20 seconds. Place the warm tortillas out and spread the mashed sweet potato evenly on each, as shown in the video.

6. Then, top each tortilla with an equal amount of scrambled eggs, diced avocado, black beans, and shredded cheese. Then, drizzle a tablespoon of enchilada sauce on each. Season with salt and pepper, if desired. Fold the ends in, then roll the burrito tightly.

7. Place the items on a baking sheet and heat in the oven at 300° for 5-10 minutes, or microwave them for one to two minutes. Serve with sour cream, Greek yogurt, salsa, or hot sauce. Makes 6 burritos. Freezer instructions are in the notes!

Notes: These burritos are freezer-friendly. Simply wrap in plastic wrap, then in foil, and place in the freezer. To warm up the food, take off the foil and plastic wrap, then microwave for approximately 2-3 minutes.

Nutrition Facts: Calories: 398 | Carbs: 54.3g | Protein: 18.1g | Fat: 13.8g

Ezekiel Bread French Toast

Serves: 2   **Prep & Cook Time:** 20mins

Ingredients:

- 4 Slices Ezekiel Bread
- 2 Eggs
- 1/2 Cup Coconut Milk or Unsweetened Almond Milk (lite or silk)
- 2 Tbsp Coconut Sugar
- 1 pkt Stevia
- 1 tsp vanilla
- Pinch Salt
- Cinnamon

Let's Get Cooking:

1. Mix all ingredients, except for the Ezekiel bread, in a large mixing bowl.
2. Dip each bread slice in the mixture; ensure both sides are thoroughly coated.
3. Cook each side in the pan for approximately 5 minutes, or until it is lightly browned.
4. Add syrup and enjoy!

Nutrition Facts/Serving: Calories: 350; Carbs: 40g; Proteins: 20g; Fats: 15g

Vegetable Hash with Poached Eggs

Serves: 4   **Prep & Cook Time:** 40mins

Ingredients:

- 2 tablespoons canola oil
- 1 medium red onion, finely diced
- 4 cups of diced vegetables (like; red pepper, carrot, celery, kohlrabi and parsnip)
- Kosher salt to taste
- 1 teaspoon cumin seeds, coarsely ground
- 2 teaspoons sweet paprika
- 2 tablespoons ketchup
- Freshly ground pepper to taste
- 4 poached eggs

Let's Get Cooking:

1. Warm the oil over medium heat in a large nonstick pan. Pour in your onion and cook, stirring frequently, until it starts to soften. Add the rest of the vegetables with a pinch of salt.

2. Continue to cook, stirring frequently, until the vegetables start to soften, which should take about five minutes.

3. Stir in the ground cumin seeds and paprika till they are well mixed with the vegetables. Keep cooking, frequently stirring for 15 minutes until the vegetables reach a crisp-tender texture. Then, add ketchup and cook for an additional five minutes.

4. Firmly press the vegetable mixture into a flat layer in the pan. Allow it to cook undisturbed for five minutes until a crust forms on the bottom. Stir the mixture, press it down once more, and cook for an

additional five minutes to form another crust. After stirring again, taste the mixture and adjust the seasoning with salt and pepper to your preference.

5. The vegetables should be completely tender and the mixture should have a nicely browned appearance with a hint of sweetness. Once achieved, take the pan off the heat.

6. Scoop the hash onto plates, make a well in the center, place a poached egg on top, and serve immediately.

Note: To poach an egg, fill a nonstick frying pan with water, one that has a tight-fitting lid (such as an omelet pan with a perfectly fitting saucepan lid), and bring it to a boil. Stir in 1 teaspoon of vinegar. Crack an egg into a teacup, then gently pour it into the boiling water. Cover the pan tightly, switch off the heat, and let it sit for four minutes. Next, lift the egg out with a slotted spoon and let it drain on a kitchen towel. If not using immediately, place the egg in a bowl of water.

Nutrition Facts/4 Servings: Calories: 211 | Fat: 12g | Carbs: 19g | Protein: 9g

Open Face Breakfast Sandwich

Serves: 8 sandwiches   **Prep & Cook Time:** 15mins

Ingredients:

- 8 hard-boiled eggs finely chopped
- 2 large celery stalk finely chopped
- 1 cup part-skim ricotta cheese
- 0.5 cup low-fat cottage cheese
- 0.5 cup pickled jalapeños finely chopped
- 4 Tablespoons pickled jalapeños juice
- Kosher salt & fresh pepper to taste
- 6 teaspoons fresh thyme chives or rosemary

Let's Get Cooking:

1. Add all the ingredients in a medium-sized bowl; 8 hard-boiled eggs, 2 large celery stalks, 1 cup part-skim ricotta cheese, 0.5 cups low fat cottage cheese, 0.5 cups pickled jalapeños, 4 Tablespoons pickled jalapeños juice, Kosher salt & fresh pepper to taste,6 teaspoons fresh thyme
2. Mix using a fork or spatula until they are well combined.
3. Add kosher salt and freshly ground pepper for taste.
4. Serve it on a toast or as a side to complement your preferred main course. Top with avocado and herbs.

Nutrition Facts/1 cup: Calories: 194 | Carbs: 20g | Protein: 14g | Fat: 7g

Turkey Bacon and Egg Breakfast Tacos

Serves: 16 tacos   **Prep and Cook Time:** 15mins

Ingredients:

- 16 small corn or flour tortillas look for street-size
- 2 tablespoon extra-virgin olive oil
- 2 can reduced-sodium black beans 15 ounces rinsed and drained
- 0.5 teaspoon garlic powder
- 0.5 teaspoon onion powder
- 0.5 teaspoon kosher salt plus a few pinches
- 0.25 teaspoon cayenne pepper
- 0.5 cup water
- 2 tablespoon unsalted butter divided
- 16 large eggs

Optional Toppings (pick at least 2):

- Shredded cheese
- Salsa
- Diced avocado
- Baked Bacon chopped
- Cilantro chopped

Let's Get Cooking:

1. Turn on your oven to 350°F and put eight tortillas wrapped in foil on a tray to warm up for 8-10 minutes. If you want to do it quicker, you can also heat them in the microwave with a wet cloth on top for 30 seconds.

2. Put some oil in a pan, then add beans and some spices. Smash the beans while they cook until they're smooth but still have some lumps.

3. Pour water into the beans and let it boil away until the beans are really smooth. Mix in some butter, taste it, and add more spices if you like. Keep it warm.

4. In a bowl, whisk eggs until they look light yellow. Then melt some butter in a frying pan over medium heat.

5. Turn down the heat, pour in the eggs, and gently stir from the edges to the middle as they start to firm up.

6. Keep cooking the eggs, stirring and breaking them up, until they're almost done but still a bit runny. Take them off the heat and stir until they're just right and soft.

7. Cooking the eggs should take about 3-5 minutes. Sprinkle some salt on them when they're cooked.

8. Make your tacos by putting beans first, then scrambled eggs, and add your favorite toppings like cheese, salsa, and avocado. Eat them right away.

Nutrition Facts (1 taco): Calories: 148; Carbs: 12g; Protein: 7g; Fat: 8g

Smoked Salmon on Whole Grain Toast

Serves: 2   **Prep and Cook Time:** 5mins

Ingredients:

- Slice of toast

- 2 tbsp cream cheese

- Salt, pepper, and lemon juice

- 4 ounces smoked salmon

- 2 teaspoon capers

- 6-8 very thin slices of red onion

Let's Get Cooking:

1. Toast your slice of bread

2. Mix cream cheese with salt, pepper & lemon juice to taste

3. Top toast with cream cheese, smoked salmon, capers, and red onions to taste

Notes: For avocado toast substitute cream cheese for 1/4 size of avocado

Nutrition Facts (1 slice): Calories: 239 | Carbs: 22g | Protein: 12g | Fat: 9g

Southwest Tofu Scramble

Serves: 2   **Prep and Cook Time:** 30mins

Ingredients:

For Scramble:

- 8 ounces extra-firm tofu
- 1-2 Tbsp olive oil
- Medium-sized red onion (thinly sliced)
- Medium-sized red bell pepper (thinly sliced)
- 2 cups kale (loosely chopped)

For Sauce:

- 1/2 tsp sea salt (reduce amount for less salty sauce)
- 1/2 tsp garlic powder
- 1/2 tsp ground cumin
- 1/4 tsp chili powder
- Water (to thin)
- 1/4 tsp turmeric (optional)
- Salsa/Cilantro/Hot Sauce (optional)
- Potatoes, Toast or Fruit

Let's Get Cooking:

1. Pat tofu dry and roll in a clean, absorbent towel with something heavy on top, such as a cast-iron pan, for 15 minutes.

2. As the tofu drains, create the sauce by combining dry spices in a small bowl and mixing in enough water to form a pourable consistency. Set aside.

3. Prepare the vegetables and heat a large pan over medium heat. When it's hot, add olive oil, onion, and red pepper. Season the mixture

with a pinch of salt and pepper, stir well. Continue to sauté the ingredients until they become soft, which usually takes around 5 minutes.

4. Add kale, season again with salt and pepper, then cover and allow to steam for two minutes.
5. Meanwhile, remove the tofu from its packaging and crumble it into bite-sized pieces using a fork.
6. Use a spatula to move the veggies to one side of the pan and add tofu. Sauté for two minutes, then add the sauce, drizzling most of it over the tofu and a bit over the vegetables. Stir immediately, evenly distributing the sauce. Continue cooking for an additional 5 to 7 minutes until the tofu is slightly browned.
7. Serve at once alongside breakfast potatoes, toast, or fruit. You can add more flavor with salsa, hot sauce, and fresh cilantro. You can also freeze it for up to one month and then reheat it on the stovetop or in the microwave.

Nutrition Facts (1 serving): Calories: 212 | Carbs: 7.1g | Protein: 16.4g | Fat: 15g

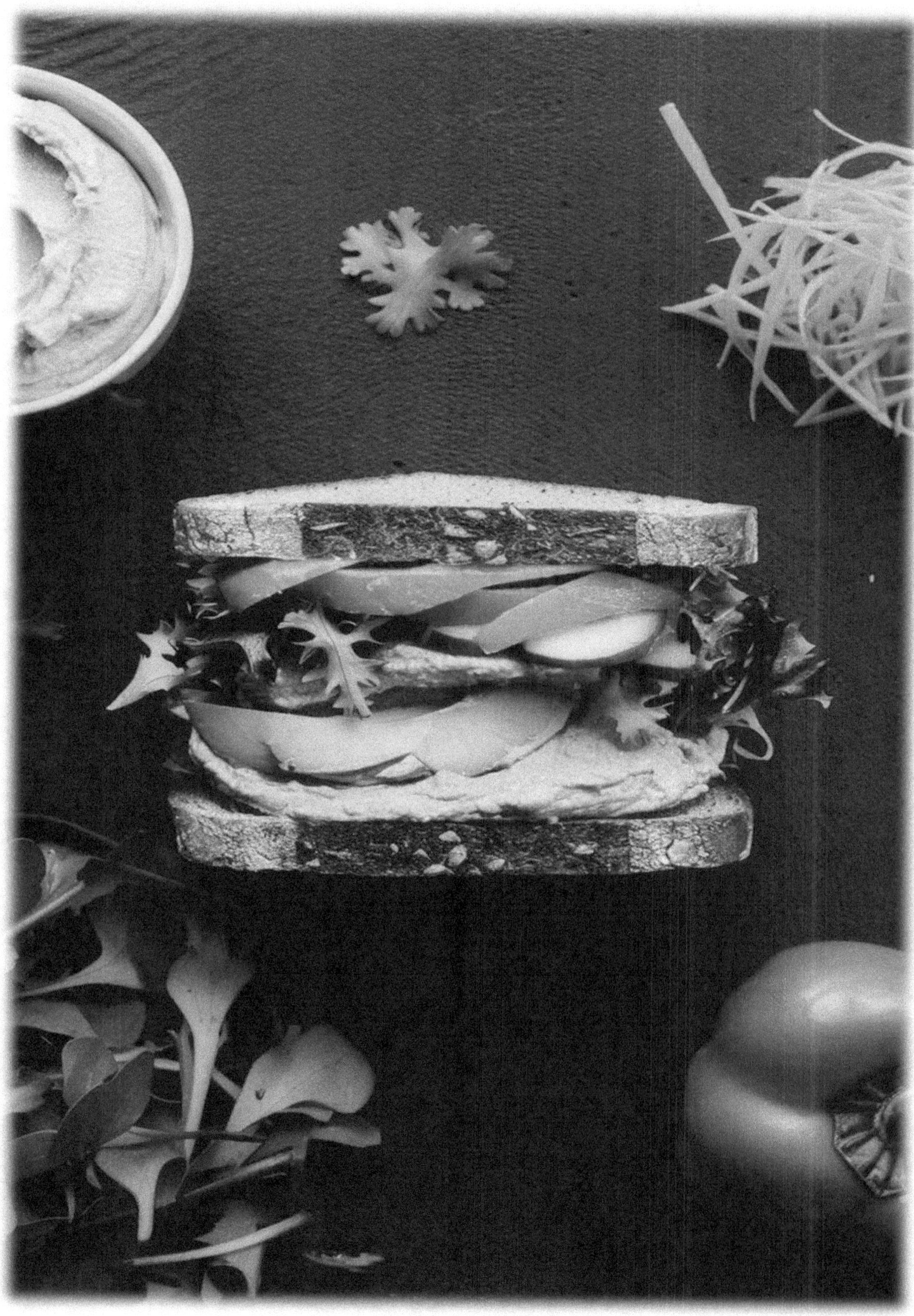

TASTEFUL LUNCH RECIPES

Chipotle-Lime Cauliflower Taco Bowls

Serves: 4   **Prep and Cook Time:** 30mins

Ingredients:

- Juice from 2 limes (around 1/4 cup)
- 1-2 tablespoons of chopped chipotle chiles in adobo sauce
- 1 tablespoon of honey
- 2 cloves of garlic
- 1/2 teaspoon of salt
- 1 small head of cauliflower, cut into bite-sized pieces
- 1 small red onion (sliced)
- 2 cups of cooked quinoa, cooled
- 1 cup of rinsed black beans
- 1/2 cup of crumbled queso fresco
- 1 cup of shredded red cabbage
- 1 ripe avocado
- 4 lime wedges (optional)

Let's Get Cooking:

1. Crank up your oven to 450°F and line a baking sheet with foil.
2. In a blender, combine the lime juice, chipotles, honey, garlic, and salt. Blend until mostly smooth.
3. In a large bowl, toss the cauliflower with the zesty sauce until well coated.
4. Spread the saucy cauliflower onto the prepared baking sheet and sprinkle the sliced onions over the top.

5. Roast for 18-20 minutes, stirring once, until the cauliflower is tender and lightly charred in spots. Set aside to cool slightly.
6. Divide the quinoa among 4 single-serve containers (1/2 cup each).
7. Top each with 1/4 of the roasted cauliflower mixture, 1/4 cup black beans, and 2 tablespoons of queso fresco.
8. Seal and refrigerate for up to 4 days.
9. Vent the lid and microwave one container for 2 1/2 to 3 minutes until steaming hot. Top with 1/4 of the shredded cabbage and sliced avocado. A squeeze of lime juice adds a bright finishing touch!

Nutrition Facts/Serving: Calories: 350 | Protein: 15g | Carbs: 45g | Fat: 15g

Veggie & Hummus Sandwich

Serves: 1   **Prep Time (No Cooking):** 10mins

Ingredients:

- 2 slices of whole-grain bread
- 3 tablespoons of hummus
- 1/4 ripe avocado, mashed
- 1/2 cup of mixed salad greens
- 1/4 red bell pepper, sliced
- 1/4 cup of sliced cucumber
- 1/4 cup of shredded carrot

Let's Get Cooking:

1. Spread one slice of bread with hummus and the other with mashed avocado.
2. Layer the greens, bell pepper slices, cucumber, and shredded carrot between the two slices.
3. Slice in half and enjoy this fresh, crunchy sandwich!

Nutrition Facts/Serving: Calories: 300 | Protein: 10g | Carbs: 40g | Fat: 10g

Spinach & Strawberry Meal-Prep Salad

Serves: 4   **Prep and Cook Time:** 27mins

Ingredients:

- 1 pound of boneless chicken thighs (skinless)
- 1/2 teaspoon of kosher salt
- 1/2 teaspoon of dried thyme
- 1/2 teaspoon of ground pepper
- 8 cups of baby spinach
- 2 cups of sliced strawberries
- 1/4 cup of crumbled feta cheese; optional
- 1/4 cup of chopped, toasted walnuts
- 6 tablespoons of store-bought balsamic vinaigrette

Let's Get Cooking:

1. Preheat your oven to 400°F and line a baking sheet with parchment or foil.
2. Season the chicken thighs with salt, thyme, and pepper, then roast for 15-17 minutes until fully cooked. Let cool it, then slice into pieces.
3. Divide the spinach among 4 single-serve containers (2 cups each). Top each with 1/4 of the sliced chicken, strawberries, feta (if using), and walnuts.
4. Ensure the salad containers are sealed and store them in the refrigerator for up to four days for keep.
5. Transfer 1 1/2 tablespoons of vinaigrette into 4 small containers and refrigerate for up to 5 days.
6. Dress your salad with the vinaigrette.

Nutrition Facts/Serving: Calories 374; Fat 24g; Carbs 14g; Protein 26g

Smoked Salmon Salad Nicoise

Serves: 2   **Prep and Cook Time:** 35mins

Ingredients:

- 8 ounces of small red potatoes, scrubbed and halved
- 6 ounces of crisp green beans (preferably; haricots verts) halved
- 2 tablespoons of reduced-fat mayonnaise
- 1 tablespoon of white wine vinegar
- 1 teaspoon of lemon juice
- 1 teaspoon of Worcestershire sauce
- 1 teaspoon of Dijon mustard
- 1/2 teaspoon of dried dill
- 1/4 teaspoon of ground black pepper
- 6 cups of mixed salad greens
- 1/2 small cucumber, halved, seeded, and thinly sliced
- 12 cherry or grape tomatoes, halved
- 4 ounces of smoked salmon, cut into 2-inch pieces

Let's Get Cooking:

1. Prepare a large bowl of ice water and set it next to the stove.
2. In a large saucepan, bring 1 inch of water to a boil.
3. Place the halved potatoes in a steamer basket over the boiling water, cover, and steam for 10-15 minutes until tender when pierced with a fork. Transfer the potatoes to the ice water using a slotted spoon.
4. Add the green beans to the steamer basket, cover, and steam for 4-5 minutes until tender-crisp. Move the beans into the ice water.
5. Drain the potatoes and beans on a towel-lined baking sheet.

6. In a large bowl, whisk together the mayonnaise, vinegar, lemon juice, Worcestershire sauce, mustard, dill, and pepper.

7. Add the potatoes, green beans, salad greens, cucumber, and tomatoes to the dressing, and gently toss to coat.

8. Divide the salad between 2 plates and top with the smoked salmon pieces.

Nutrition Facts/Serving: Calories: 400 | Protein: 25g | Fat: 15g | Carbs: 45g

Sweet Potato, Kale & Chicken Salad with Peanut Dressing

Serves: 4   **Prep & Cook Time:** 35mins

Ingredients:

For the Salad:

- Two medium sweet potatoes, diced into cubes.
- 1 1/2 teaspoons extra-virgin olive oil
- 1/4 teaspoon of kosher salt
- 1/8 teaspoon of ground pepper
- 6 cups of chopped curly kale
- 2 cups of cooked chicken breast (shredded)
- 1/4 cup of chopped unsalted peanuts

For the Peanut Dressing:

- half cup of smooth, unsweetened natural peanut butter
- 1/4 cup of reduced-sodium tamari or soy sauce
- 1/4 cup of fresh lime juice
- 2 tablespoons of water
- 1 tablespoon of honey
- 1 teaspoon of minced garlic

Let's Get Cooking:

1. Preheat your oven to 425°F and line a rimmed baking sheet with foil, lightly coated with cooking spray.
2. In a large bowl, toss the sweet potato cubes with olive oil, salt, and pepper.
3. Arrange the sweet potatoes in a single layer on the prepared baking sheet and roast for about 20 minutes, turning once, until tender and lightly browned.
4. Transfer 2 tablespoons of the peanut dressing into each of 4 small lidded containers and refrigerate for up to 4 days.
5. Divide the chopped kale among 4 single-serve containers (about 1 1/2 cups each).
6. Top each container with one-fourth of the roasted sweet potatoes and 1/2 cup of shredded chicken.
7. Seal the containers and refrigerate for up to 4 days.
8. In a jar, whisk together the peanut butter, tamari (or soy sauce), lime juice, water, honey, and garlic for the dressing.
9. Just before serving, drizzle each salad with a portion of the peanut dressing and toss well to coat.
10. Top with 1 tablespoon of chopped peanuts for a delightful crunch!

Nutrition Facts/Serving: Calories: 400 | Protein: 25g | Carbs: 40g | Fat: 15g

Meal-Prep Vegan Lettuce Wraps

Serves: 4   **Prep & Cook Time:** 25mins

Ingredients:

- 4 servings of crispy tofu
- 2 heads of iceberg lettuce, separated into leaves
- 1/4 red cabbage, thinly sliced
- 1 cup of kimchi
- 2 green onions, diced
- 1/2 cup of crispy fried noodles
- 4 tablespoons of hoisin sauce
- 3 tablespoons of crushed peanuts
- 3 tablespoons of sesame seeds

For the Tahini Chili Dressing:

- 4 tablespoons of tahini
- 2 tablespoons of water
- 2 tablespoons of sweet chili sauce

Let's Get Wrapping:

1. Start by making the crispy tofu and preparing the tahini chili dressing according to the recipes.
2. Carefully separate the iceberg lettuce leaves from the root, creating wraps.
3. Load each lettuce wrap with a generous spoonful of crispy tofu, a splash of tahini chili dressing, some kimchi, red cabbage, green onions, crispy noodles, crushed peanuts, sesame seeds, and finish with a dollop of hoisin sauce.

4. Enjoy these flavorful and crunchy wraps immediately for the ultimate fresh and satisfying meal!

Nutrition Facts/Serving: Calories: 194.1 | Carbs: 20.2g | Protein: 5.1g | Fat: 11.6g

Mason Jar Power Salad with Chickpeas & Tuna

Serves: 1   **Prep and Cook Time**: 25mins

Ingredients:

- 1 clove of garlic, minced
- 1 tablespoon of white wine vinegar
- 1 1/2 teaspoons of Dijon mustard (your choice of coarse or smooth)
- 1/2 teaspoon of honey
- 1/8 teaspoon of salt
- Freshly ground black pepper, to taste
- 1/3 cup of extra-virgin oil (olive or canola)
- 3 cups of bite-sized chopped kale
- 1 (2.5-ounce) pouch of tuna in water
- 1/2 cup of canned chickpeas, rinsed
- 1 medium carrot, shredded

Let's Get Layering:

1. Start by whisking together the garlic, vinegar, mustard, honey, salt, and a generous grind of pepper in a small bowl. Slowly drizzle in the oil while whisking continuously to create delightful vinaigrette.
2. In a separate bowl, toss the chopped kale with 2 tablespoons of the vinaigrette until well coated.
3. Layer the dressed kale into a 1-quart mason jar.

4. Top the kale with the tuna, chickpeas, and shredded carrot.

5. Screw the lid on tightly, and your salad is ready to go! Refrigerate for up to 2 days.

6. When you're ready to enjoy, simply empty the jar contents into a bowl and give it a good toss to combine all the flavors.

Nutrition Facts/Serving: Calories: 800 | Protein: 30g | Fat: 60g | Carbs: 35g

8. *Winter Kale & Quinoa Salad with Avocado*

Serves: 2   **Prep and Cook Time:** 40mins

Ingredients:

- 1 small sweet potato (peeled and cut into cube pieces)
- 2 1/2 teaspoons of olive oil, divided
- 1/2 avocado
- 1 tablespoon of fresh lime juice
- 1 clove of garlic, peeled
- 1/2 teaspoon of ground cumin
- 1/8 teaspoon of salt
- 1/8 teaspoon of ground pepper
- 1-2 tablespoons of water
- 1 cup of cooked quinoa
- 3/4 cup of rinsed, no-salt-added canned black beans
- 1 1/2 cups of chopped baby kale
- 2 tablespoons of pepitas (pumpkin seeds)
- 1 scallion, chopped

Let's Get Cooking:

1. Preheat your oven to 400°F.

2. Toss the sweet potato cubes with 1 teaspoon of olive oil on a large rimmed baking sheet, and roast for about 25 minutes, stirring once halfway, until tender.

3. Meanwhile, in a blender or food processor, combine the remaining 1 1/2 teaspoons of olive oil, avocado, lime juice, garlic, cumin, salt, pepper, and 1 tablespoon of water. Process until smooth, adding another tablespoon of water if needed to reach your desired consistency.

4. In a medium bowl, combine the roasted sweet potato, quinoa, black beans, and baby kale.

5. Drizzle the avocado dressing over the salad and gently toss to coat everything evenly.

6. Top with the crunchy pepitas and chopped scallion for a delightful finishing touch.

Nutrition Facts/Serving: Calories: 400 | Protein: 15g | Carbs: 40g | Fat: 15g

Vegan Superfood Grain Bowls

Serves: 4   **Prep & Cook Time:** 30mins

Ingredients:

- 1 (8-ounce) pouch of microwavable quinoa
- 1/2 cup of hummus
- 2 tablespoons of fresh lemon juice
- 1 (5-ounce) package of baby kale
- 1 package of refrigerated cooked whole baby beets (sliced) or 2 cups from the salad bar
- 1 cup of edamame (thawed and shelled)
- 1 medium avocado, sliced
- 1/4 cup of unsalted toasted sunflower seeds

Let's Get Cooking:

1. Cook the quinoa as directed on the packaging, then allow it to cool.
2. Combine the hummus and lemon juice in a small bowl. Thin it out with a splash of water until you reach your desired dressing consistency. Divide the dressing into four small condiment containers with lids and place them in the refrigerator.
3. Divide the baby kale among 4 single-serve containers with lids.
4. Layer each container with half a cup of cooked quinoa, half a cup of sliced beets, a quarter cup of edamame, and a tablespoon of sunflower seeds.
5. When you're ready to enjoy, top each bowl with 1/4 of the sliced avocado and drizzle with the hummus dressing.

Nutrition Facts/Serving: Calories: 350 | Protein: 15g | Carbs: 40g | Fat: 15g

Tomato, Cucumber & White-Bean Salad with Basil Vinaigrette

Serves: 4   **Prep and Cook Time:**

Ingredients:

For the Basil Vinaigrette:

- half cup of packed fresh basil
- 1/4 cup of extra-virgin olive oil
- 3 tablespoons of red wine vinegar
- 1 tablespoon of finely chopped shallot
- 2 teaspoons of Dijon mustard
- 1 teaspoon of honey
- 1/4 teaspoon of salt
- 1/4 teaspoon of ground pepper

For the Salad:

- 10 cups of mixed salad greens
- 1 can of low-sodium cannellini beans, rinsed
- 1 cup of cherry or grape tomatoes (halved)
- 1/2 cucumber, halved lengthwise and sliced (about 1 cup)

Let's Get Cooking:

1. Combine the basil, olive oil, vinegar, shallot, mustard, honey, salt, and pepper in a mini food processor. Process until mostly smooth, creating a flavorful basil vinaigrette.

2. Transfer the vinaigrette to a large bowl and add the mixed greens, cannellini beans, tomatoes, and sliced cucumber.

3. Gently toss everything together until the salad is evenly coated with the delicious basil vinaigrette.

Chimichurri Noodle Bowls

Serves: 4   **Prep and Cook Time:** 40mins

Ingredients:

For the Chimichurri Sauce:

- 2 cups of fresh flat-leaf parsley
- 5 cloves of garlic
- 3 tablespoons of lemon juice
- 1 tablespoon of fresh oregano
- 1/2 teaspoon of crushed red pepper (optional)
- 1/2 teaspoon of salt
- 1/4 teaspoon of ground black pepper
- 1/2 cup of extra-virgin olive oil

For the Noodle Bowls:

- 4 ounces of whole-grain spaghetti
- 8 cups of zucchini noodles (from about 3 medium zucchini)
- 12 ounces of peeled, cooked shrimp
- 1/4 cup of crumbled feta cheese

Let's Get Cooking:

1. Boil a large pot of water for the pasta.
2. Prepare the chimichurri sauce by blending the parsley, garlic, lemon juice, oregano, crushed red pepper (if using), salt, and black pepper in a food processor until smooth. With the motor running, slowly drizzle in the olive oil until well combined.

3. Set aside 2 tablespoons of the chimichurri sauce into each of 4 small lidded containers and refrigerate. Store any remaining sauce separately for another use.

4. Cook the spaghetti according to package instructions, drain, rinse with cold water, and transfer to a large bowl. Add the zucchini noodles and gently toss everything together using tongs or two large forks.

5. Divide the noodle mixture among 4 lidded single-serve containers, and top each with 3 ounces of shrimp and 1 tablespoon of crumbled feta.

6. Seal the containers and refrigerate for up to 4 days.

7. When you're ready to enjoy, simply toss the noodle bowl with the chilled chimichurri sauce just before serving.

Nutrition Facts/Serving: Calories: 400 | Protein: 25g | Carbs: 40g | Fat: 20g

White Bean & Veggie Salad

Serves: 1   **Prep Time (No Cooking):** 10mins

Ingredients:

-   2 cups of mixed salad greens
-   3/4 cup of veggies (chopped cucumbers & cherry tomatoes)
-   1/3 cup of canned white beans, rinsed and drained
-   1/2 avocado, diced
-   1 tablespoon of red wine vinegar
-   2 teaspoons of extra-virgin olive oil
-   1/4 teaspoon of kosher salt
-   Freshly ground black pepper, to taste

Let's Get Cooking:

1. In a medium bowl, combine the mixed greens, chopped veggies, white beans, and diced avocado.
2. Drizzle the vinegar and olive oil over the salad.
3. Season with salt and a few grinds of black pepper.
4. Carefully stir all the ingredients until they are well mixed.
5. Transfer the salad to a large plate and enjoy this simple, yet flavorful and nourishing meal!

Nutrition Facts/Serving: Calories: 300 | Protein: 10g | Carbs: 20g | Fat: 15g

Lemon-Roasted Vegetable Hummus Bowls

Serves: 4   **Prep and Cook Time:** 40mins

Ingredients:

- 1 1/2 cups of cauliflower florets
- 1 1/2 cups of broccoli florets
- 2 cloves of garlic, thinly sliced
- 1 tablespoon of extra-virgin olive oil
- 1 teaspoon of dried oregano
- 1/4 teaspoon of salt
- 3/4 cup of diced red bell pepper (1-inch pieces)
- 3/4 cup of diced zucchini (1-inch pieces)
- 2 teaspoons of lemon zest
- 2 cups of cooked tri-color quinoa, cooled
- 1 cup of hummus
- 4 lemon wedges
- 1 medium avocado

Let's Get Cooking:

1. Preheat your oven to 425°F.
2. Combine the cauliflower, broccoli, and sliced garlic on a rimmed baking sheet. Drizzle olive oil over the dish and season with oregano and salt to taste. Toss to mix.
3. Roast for 10 minutes, then add the diced bell pepper and zucchini to the baking sheet. Stir to combine and roast for another 10-15 minutes, or until the veggies are crisp-tender and lightly browned.
4. Sprinkle the lemon zest over the roasted veggies and set aside to cool slightly before assembling the bowls.

5. Divide the roasted veggies among 4 single-serve containers, and top each with 1/2 cup of quinoa and 1/4 cup of hummus. Place a lemon wedge into each container.

6. Seal the containers and refrigerate for up to 4 days.

7. Squeeze the lemon wedge over the bowl and top with diced avocado for a creamy, zingy finish!

Nutrition Facts/Serving: Calories: 360 | Fat: 19g | Carbs: 40g | Protein: 12g

Mixed Greens with Lentils & Sliced Apple

Serves: 1   **Prep Time (No Cooking):** 10mins

Ingredients:

- 1 1/2 cups of mixed salad greens
- 1/2 cup of cooked lentils
- 1 apple, cored and sliced (divided)
- 1 1/2 tablespoons of crumbled feta cheese
- 1 tablespoon of red wine vinegar
- 2 teaspoons of extra-virgin olive oil

Let's Assemble:

1. In a bowl or on a plate, arrange the mixed greens.

2. Top the greens with the cooked lentils, about half of the sliced apples, and the crumbled feta cheese.

3. Drizzle the red wine vinegar and olive oil over the salad.

4. Serve with the remaining apple slices on the side for a refreshing and crunchy addition.

Nutrition Info (serving): Calories: 300 | Protein: 15g | Carbs: 30g | Fat: 10g

Rainbow Grain Bowl with Cashew Tahini Sauce

Serves: 1   **Prep and Cook Time:** 1hour

Ingredients:

For the Cashew Tahini Sauce:

- 3/4 cup of unsalted cashews
- 1/2 cup of water
- 1/4 cup of packed parsley leaves
- 1 tbsp of lemon juice or cider vinegar
- 1 tablespoon of extra-virgin olive oil
- 1/2 teaspoon of reduced-sodium tamari or soy sauce (gluten-free)
- 1/4 teaspoon of salt

For the Rainbow Bowl:

- 1/2 cup of cooked lentils
- 1/2 cup of cooked quinoa
- 1/2 cup of shredded red cabbage
- 1/4 cup of grated raw beet
- 1/4 cup of chopped bell pepper
- 1/4 cup of grated carrot
- 1/4 cup of sliced cucumber
- 1 tablespoon of toasted chopped cashews (for garnish)

Let's Get Cooking:

1. Combine the cashews, water, parsley leaves, lemon juice (or vinegar), olive oil, tamari (or soy sauce), and salt in your blender. Blend until smooth and creamy, creating the cashew tahini sauce.

2. Place the cooked lentils and quinoa in a shallow serving bowl.

3. Arrange the shredded red cabbage, grated beet, chopped bell pepper, grated carrot, and sliced cucumber around the lentils and quinoa, creating a vibrant rainbow of colors.

4. Spoon 2 tablespoons of the cashew tahini sauce over the top of the bowl (save any extra sauce for another use).

5. Garnish with the toasted chopped cashews for a delightful crunch.

Nutrition Facts/Serving: Calories: 361 | Fat: 10g | Carbs: 54g | Protein: 17g

DINNER RECIPES

Chickpea Pasta with Mushrooms & Kale

Serves: 4   **Prep and Cook Time:** 30mins

Ingredients:

- 8 ounces of chickpea rotini or penne pasta
- 1/4 cup of extra-virgin olive oil
- 2 large cloves of garlic, sliced
- A pinch of crushed red pepper
- 8 cups of chopped fresh kale
- 8 ounces of cremini mushrooms, quartered
- 1/2 teaspoon of dried thyme
- 1/2 teaspoon of salt
- Grated Parmesan cheese for serving (optional)

Let's Get Cooking:

1. Prepare the chickpea pasta following the instructions on the package, drain when done. Set aside one cup of water.

2. Warm the olive oil in a large pan on medium heat. Add the sliced garlic and crushed red pepper, and sauté for about 1 minute, allowing the aromas to release.

3. Add the chopped kale, quartered mushrooms, dried thyme, and salt to the pan. Cook for about 5 minutes, stirring occasionally, until the vegetables are tender and soft.

4. Stir in the cooked pasta and enough of the reserved cooking water to create a luscious sauce. Cook for an additional minute, stirring continuously, until everything is combined and heated through.

5. Serve hot, topped with grated Parmesan cheese if you like.

Nutrition Facts/serving: Calories: 350 | Protein: 15g | Fat: 14g | Carbs: 45g

Sheet-Pan Chili-Lime Salmon with Potatoes & Peppers

Serves: 4   **Prep and Cook Time:** 40mins

Ingredients:

1 pound of Yukon Gold potatoes, cut into 3/4-inch pieces

2 tablespoons of extra-virgin olive oil

3/4 teaspoon of salt, divided

1/4 teaspoon of ground black pepper

2 teaspoons of chili powder

1 teaspoon of ground cumin

1/2 teaspoon of garlic powder

1 lime, zested and quartered

2 medium bell peppers (sliced)

1 1/4 pounds of center-cut salmon fillet (cut into 4 portions)

Let's Get Roasting:

1. Preheat your oven to 425ºF and coat a large-rimmed baking sheet with cooking spray.

2. Toss the potato pieces with 1 tablespoon of olive oil, 1/4 teaspoon of salt, and ground black pepper In a medium bowl. Spread the potatoes onto the prepared baking sheet and roast for 15 minutes.

3. Combine the chili powder, cumin, garlic powder, lime zest, and the remaining 1/2 teaspoon of salt In a small bowl.

4. Place the sliced bell peppers in the medium bowl and add the remaining 1 tablespoon of olive oil and 1/2 tablespoon of the spice mixture. Toss to coat the peppers evenly.
5. Coat the salmon with the remaining spice mixture.
6. After 15 minutes, remove the baking sheet from the oven and add the seasoned bell peppers to the potatoes, stirring to combine.
7. Roast for another 5 minutes, then remove the pan from the oven.
8. Move some of the vegetables aside and add the spiced salmon to the pan.
9. Return the pan to the oven and roast for an additional 6-8 minutes, or until the salmon is just cooked through.
10. Serve hot, with a squeeze of fresh lime juice from the quartered limes.

Nutrition Facts/serving: Calories: 450 | Protein: 30g | Fat: 20g | Carbs: 40gr

Pork Paprikash with Cauliflower Rice

Serves: 4   **Prep and Cook Time:** 45mins

Ingredients:

- 1 (1 pound) natural pork tenderloin
- 6 cups of chopped cauliflower (about 1 1/2 pounds)
- 2 tablespoons of olive oil, divided
- 1/8 teaspoon of salt, plus 1/4 teaspoon
- 1 medium onion (cut into thin slices)
- 1 1/2 tablespoons of paprika, plus more for garnish (optional)
- 1/2 teaspoon of ground black pepper
- 1 can of no-salt-added diced tomatoes with basil, garlic & oregano
- 1 cup of reduced-sodium chicken broth
- 1/4 cup of finely chopped mild banana peppers
- 1/3 cup of light sour cream (optional)
- 2 tablespoons of all-purpose flour
- 8 teaspoons of light sour cream (optional)

Let's Get Cooking:

1. Trim any excess fat from the pork tenderloin and cut it into bite-sized pieces. Set aside.
2. Place the chopped cauliflower in a food processor and pulse several times until it resembles rice-sized pieces.
3. Heat one tablespoon of olive oil in a large nonstick pan over medium-high heat. Add the cauliflower "rice" and 1/8 teaspoon of salt. Cook for 8-10 minutes, stirring occasionally, until golden brown flecks appear throughout.

4. In another large pan, heat the remaining 1 tablespoon of olive oil over medium-high heat. Add the pork pieces and onion wedges, and cook for about 3 minutes, stirring occasionally, until the meat starts to brown.

5. Sprinkle the pork and onions with 1 1/2 tablespoons of paprika, ground black pepper, and the remaining 1/4 teaspoon of salt. Continue cooking and stirring for one additional minute.

6. Add the canned diced tomatoes (with their juices), chicken broth, and chopped banana peppers to the pork mixture. Boil well, then reduce the heat to medium-low, cover, and simmer for 5 minutes.

7. Increase the heat to medium-high and cook, uncovered, for 4-6 minutes, stirring frequently, until the sauce thickens slightly.

8. Whisk together 1/3 cup of light sour cream (if using) and the all-purpose flour in a small bowl. Stir this mixture into the pork and continue cooking until the sauce thickens and bubbles.

9. Present the Pork Paprikash atop the cauliflower "rice." Optionally, top each portion with two teaspoons of light sour cream and a dash of paprika for garnish.

Nutrition Facts/serving: Calories: 319 | Fat: 12g | Carbs: 24g | Protein: 31g

One-Pot Garlicky Shrimp & Spinach

Serves: 4   **Prep and Cook Time:** 25mins

Ingredients:

- 3 tablespoons of extra-virgin olive oil
- 6 medium cloves of garlic, sliced
- 1 pound of fresh spinach
- 1 teaspoon of salt
- 1 tablespoon of lemon juice
- 1 pound of shrimp (21-30 count), peeled and deveined
- 1/4 teaspoon of crushed red pepper
- 1 tablespoon of chopped parsley
- 1 1/2 teaspoons of lemon zest

Let's Get Cooking:

1. Heat 1 tablespoon of olive oil over medium heat in a large pot. Add half of the sliced garlic and cook for 1-2 minutes, until it starts to brown and release its aroma.

2. Add the spinach and 1/4 teaspoon of salt to the pot, and toss to coat the leaves with the garlic-infused oil. Cook for 3-5 minutes, stirring occasionally, until the spinach is mostly wilted.

3. Take the pot off the heat and mix in the lemon juice. Transfer the wilted spinach to a bowl and keep it warm.

4. Increase the heat to medium-high and add the remaining 2 tablespoons of olive oil to the pot. Add the remaining sliced garlic and cook for another 1-2 minutes, until it starts to brown.

5. Add the shrimp, crushed red pepper, and the remaining 1/8 teaspoon of salt to the pot. Cook for 3-5 minutes, stirring continuously, until the shrimp are just cooked through and opaque.

6. Serve the garlicky shrimp over the wilted spinach, and garnish with lemon zest and freshly chopped parsley.

Nutrition Facts/Serving: Calories: 300 | Protein: 28g | Fat: 20g | Carbs: 8g

Beef & Bean Sloppy Joes

Serves: 4   **Prep and Cook Time:** 30mins

Ingredients:
- 1 tablespoon of extra-virgin olive oil
- 12 ounces of 90%-lean ground beef
- 1 cup of black beans (no salt included)
- 1 cup of chopped onion
- 2 tsp of New Mexico chile powder
- 1/2 teaspoon of garlic powder
- 1/2 teaspoon of onion powder
- A pinch of cayenne pepper
- 1 cup of tomato sauce (no salt included)
- 3 tablespoons of ketchup
- 1 tablespoon of reduced-sodium Worcestershire sauce
- 2 teaspoons of spicy brown mustard
- 1 teaspoon of light brown sugar
- 4 whole-wheat hamburger buns

Let's Get Cooking:

1. Heat the olive oil in a large nonstick pan on medium-high heat. Add the ground beef and cook, breaking it up with a wooden spoon, until lightly browned but not fully cooked through about 3-4 minutes. Using a slotted spoon, transfer the browned beef to a medium bowl, reserving the drippings in the pan.

2. Add the black beans and chopped onion to the pan with the drippings. Cook for approximately five minutes, stirring frequently, until the onion has softened.

3. Sprinkle in the chile powder, garlic powder, onion powder, and a pinch of cayenne pepper. Cook for an additional 30 seconds, stirring constantly, to release the aromas.

4. Stir in the tomato sauce, ketchup, Worcestershire sauce, spicy brown mustard, and brown sugar. Return the browned beef to the pan, and bring the mixture to a simmer.

5. Cook for about 5 minutes, stirring often, until the beef is just cooked through and the sauce has thickened slightly.

6. Toast the whole-wheat hamburger buns, and serve the sloppy joe mixture on top, piled high and ready to enjoy!

Nutrition Facts/Serving: Calories: 400 | Protein: 30g | Fat: 15g | Carbs: 40g

Seared Scallops with White Bean Ragu & Charred Lemon

Serves: 4   **Prep and Cook Time:** 30mins

Ingredients:

- 3 teaspoons of extra-virgin olive oil
- 1 pound of mature spinach or white chard, trimmed and thinly sliced
- 2 cloves of garlic, minced
- 1 tablespoon of capers, rinsed and chopped
- 1/2 teaspoon of ground pepper, divided
- 1 (15 ounce) can of no-salt-added cannellini beans, drained & rinsed
- 1 cup of low-sodium chicken broth
- 1/3 cup of dry white wine
- 1 tablespoon of butter
- 1 pound of dry sea scallops, tough side muscle removed
- 1 lemon, halved
- 2 tablespoons of chopped fresh parsley

Let's Get Cooking:

1. In a large pan, heat 2 teaspoons of olive oil over medium-high heat. Add the sliced greens and cook, stirring often, for about 4 minutes until wilted.
2. Stir in the minced garlic, chopped capers, and 1/4 teaspoon of pepper. Cook for an additional 30 seconds, stirring occasionally, until fragrant.
3. Add the cannellini beans, chicken broth, and white wine to the pan, and bring the mixture to a simmer. Reduce the heat to maintain a low simmer, cover, and cook for 5 minutes.
4. Remove the pan from heat, stir in the butter, and cover to keep warm.

5. In the meantime, season the scallops with the remaining quarter teaspoon of pepper.

6. In a separate large nonstick pan, heat the remaining 1 teaspoon of olive oil over medium-high heat. Add the seasoned scallops and cook for about 4 minutes total, turning once, until browned on both sides.

7. Transfer the seared scallops to a clean plate, and add the lemon halves to the same pan, cut-side down. Cook for about 2 minutes, until the lemon is charred.

8. Cut the charred lemon into wedges, and sprinkle the scallops and the white bean ragu with chopped fresh parsley.

9. Serve the seared scallops alongside the flavorful white bean ragu, and enjoy with the charred lemon wedges for a bright, zesty finish.

Nutrition Facts/Serving: Calories: 255 | Fat: 8g | Carbs: 21g | Protein : 21g

Power Up with this Nutrient-Packed Chopped Salad

Serves: 4   **Prep and Cook Time:** 60mins

Ingredients:

For the Salad:

- 1 lb salmon fillet
- 8 cups chopped curly kale
- 2 cups chopped broccoli
- 2 cups chopped red cabbage
- 2 cups finely diced carrots
- 1/2 cup toasted sunflower seeds

For the Dreamy Dressing:

- 1/2 cup low-fat plain yogurt
- 1/4 cup mayonnaise
- 2 tbsp lemon juice
- 2 tbsp grated parmesan
- 1 tbsp chopped fresh parsley
- 1 tbsp snipped fresh chives
- 2 tsp low-sodium tamari
- 1 clove garlic, minced
- 1/4 tsp ground pepper

Let's Get Cooking:

1. Preheat your oven's broiler and line a baking sheet with foil. Place the salmon fillet skin-side down and broil for 8-12 minutes until opaque in the center. Let cool slightly and cut into 4 portions.

2. Make the dressing by whisking together the yogurt, mayo, lemon, parmesan, herbs, tamari, garlic, and pepper.

3. In a large bowl, toss the kale, broccoli, cabbage, carrots, and sunflower seeds with 3/4 cup of the dressing until fully coated.

4. Divide the dressed salad between 4 plates or shallow bowls. Top each with a piece of the broiled salmon and an extra drizzle of the remaining dressing.

Nutrition Facts/Serving: Calories: 450 | Protein: 32g | Fat: 30g | Carbs: 25g

Nutrient-Packed Quinoa Power Bowl

Servings: 2   **Prep and Cook Time:** 45mins

Ingredients:

- 2/3 cup water
- 1/3 cup quinoa
- 1/4 tsp coarse salt
- 1 garlic clove, crushed
- 2 tsp lemon zest
- 3 tbsp lemon juice
- 3 tbsp olive oil
- 1/4 tsp pepper
- 1 cup rinsed canned chickpeas
- 1 medium carrot (shredded)
- 1/2 avocado, diced
- 5 oz package mixed greens (about 8 cups)

Let's Get Cooking:

1. Cook the quinoa according to package instructions by bringing the water to a boil, adding quinoa, covering, and simmering for 15 minutes until liquid is absorbed. Fluff the mixture with a fork and allow it to cool down a bit.
2. Make the zesty dressing by mashing the garlic with salt into a paste, then whisking in the lemon zest, juice, oil, and pepper. Reserve 3 tbsp for the greens.
3. Gently toss chickpeas, shredded carrot, avocado, and quinoa with the remaining dressing in a bowl. et it marinate for 5 mins to soak up all that flavor.
4. Place mixed greens in a large bowl and toss with the reserved 3 tbsp dressing.
5. Divide greens between two plates or bowls and top with the quinoa-chickpea mixture.

Nutrition Facts/Serving: Calories: 501 | Fat: 32g | Carbs: 47g | Protein: 12g

Summer Veggie & Egg Scramble

Serves: 4   **Prep and Cook Time:** 30mins

Ingredients:

- 1 tablespoon Olive oil
- 2 Baby potatoes, thinly sliced
- 4 cups of mixed veggies like mushrooms, bell peppers, zucchini
- 2 Scallions, chopped (white and green parts separated)
- 1 teaspoon Fresh herbs like rosemary or thyme, chopped
- 6 eggs (or a mix of 4 eggs + 4 egg whites)
- 2 cups Baby spinach or baby kale
- Salt and pepper to taste (optional)

Let's Get Cooking:

1. Sauté the potato slices in olive oil until they're starting to soften up.
2. Add the sliced veggies and the white part of the scallions. Cook the ingredients until they are tender and have a light brown color.
3. Make a well in the center and crack in the eggs. Add the scallion greens and herbs.
4. Scramble the eggs gently, pulling in the veggies from the sides as they cook.
5. Once the eggs are softly scrambled, fold in the greens—season with salt and pepper.

Nutrition Facts/Serving: Calories: 250 | Protein: 20g | Carbs: 18g | Fat: 12g

Chipotle Chicken Quinoa Burrito Bowls

Serves: 4   **Prep and Cook Time:** 40mins

Ingredients:

- 2 chipotle peppers in adobo sauce, finely chopped
- 2 tablespoons olive oil
- 1 teaspoon garlic powder
- 1 teaspoon cumin
- 4 boneless, skinless chicken breasts
- 1/2 teaspoon salt
- 2 cups cooked quinoa
- 2 cups shredded romaine lettuce
- 1 can (15 oz) pinto beans, drained and rinsed
- 1 diced avocado
- 1 cup salsa or pico de gallo
- 1/2 cup shredded cheese (such as cheddar or Monterey Jack)
- 4 lime wedges

Let's Get Cooking:

1. Make a quick chipotle glaze by mixing the peppers, olive oil, garlic, cumin. Season the chicken with salt.
2. Grill or broil the chicken, basting with the glaze during the last few minutes.
3. Once cooked, chop or shred the chipotle chicken.
4. Time to assemble! Start with quinoa in the bottom of a bowl. Top with chicken, lettuce, beans, avocado, salsa and cheese.
5. Squeeze a lime wedge over the top for bright, zesty flavor.

Nutrition Facts/Serving: Calories: 452 | Fat: 19g | Carbs: 36g | Protein: 36g

Sizzling Beef & Baby Bok Choy Stir-Fry

Serves: 4   **Prep and Cook Time:** 25mins

Ingredients:

- 1 lb flank steak, thinly sliced
- 2 tablespoons fresh ginger, minced
- 3 tablespoons soy sauce
- 2 tablespoons dry sherry
- 1 tablespoon cornstarch
- 1 teaspoon sesame oil
- 2 tablespoons oyster sauce
- 2 tablespoons vegetable oil
- 1 lb baby bok choy, trimmed and cut into pieces
- 1/2 cup chicken broth

Let's Get Cooking:

1. Marinate the beef with soy sauce, sherry, and cornstarch.
2. Fry the marinated beef in a hot wok or pan until lightly browned on the outside but still pink inside.
3. Remove beef and cook the bok choy with a splash of broth until bright green and tender-crisp.
4. Return the beef to the pan and toss everything together with a sauce made from oyster sauce and sherry.

Nutrition Facts/Serving: Calories: 363 | Carbs: 23g | Protein: 28g | Fat: 18g

Pan-Seared Steak with Crispy Herb Salad

Serves: 4   **Prep and Cook Time:** 22mins

Ingredients:

- 1 pound sirloin steak, about 1/2 inch thick
- ½ teaspoon salt, divided
- ½ teaspoon ground pepper, divided
- 2 tablespoons grapeseed oil or canola oil
- 4 cloves garlic, crushed
- 5 sprigs fresh thyme
- 3 sprigs fresh sage
- 1 sprig fresh rosemary
- 16 cups chopped escarole (about 1 pound)

Let's Get Cooking:

1. Put a little salt and pepper on the steak.
2. Get a big cast-iron pan very hot.
3. Put the steak in the pan and cook one side until it has char marks, around 3 minutes.
4. Flip the steak over and add oil, garlic, thyme, sage, and rosemary to the pan.
5. Keep cooking, stirring the herbs sometimes, until a food thermometer in the thickest part of the steak reads 125°F for medium-rare doneness, 3 to 4 more minutes.
6. Move the steak to a plate and put the garlic and herbs on top. Cover loosely with foil.
7. Add the escarole greens and a little more salt and pepper to the pan.

8. Cook while stirring often until the escarole starts to get soft, around 2 minutes.

9. Thinly slice the steak and serve with the wilted escarole greens and crispy herbs.

Nutrition Facts/Serving: Calories: 244 | Fat: 12g | Carbs; 10g | Protein: 26g

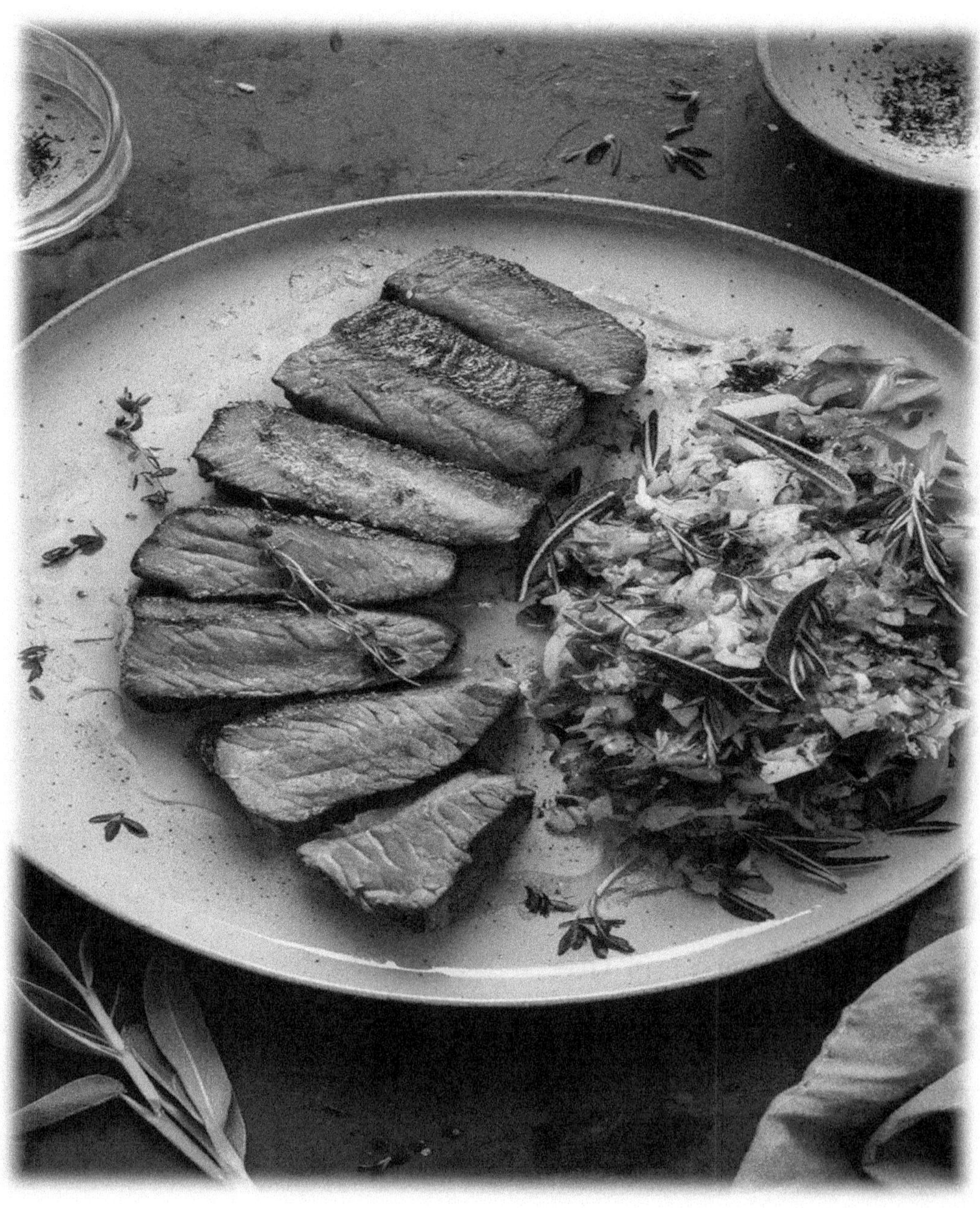

SNACKS AND SIDES

Chewy, Nutty Apricot Granola Bars

Serves: 18   **Prep and Cook Time:** 40mins

Ingredients:

- 44 grams Dried Apricots, chopped
- 1/4 cup Honey
- 2 Tablespoons Almond Butter
- 1 Tablespoon Almond Flour
- 3/4 teaspoon Salt
- 1 1/2 Tablespoons Water

Let's Get Cooking:

1. Preheat your oven and line a baking pan with parchment paper for easy removal later.
2. In a big bowl, toss together the oats, cereal, apricots, pepitas, sunflower seeds and salt.
3. In a separate bowl, microwave the brown rice syrup with the sunflower seed butter and cinnamon until melted and fragrant.
4. Pour the warm syrup mixture into the dry ingredients and stir until everything is evenly coated.
5. Firmly press the mixture into the pan that has been prepared.
6. Bake for 20-25 minutes if you want chewy bars or 30-35 minutes for a crunchier texture.
7. Let the bars cool completely before slicing into squares.

Nutrition Facts/Serving: Calories: 205 | Carbs: 33g | Protein: 4g | Fat: 8 g

Classic Greek Tahini Dip

Serves: 8   **Prep Time (No Cooking):** 15mins

Ingredients:

- 1/2 cup tahini
- 2 tablespoons lemon juice
- 1 tablespoon extra-virgin olive oil, plus more for garnish
- 1 clove garlic, crushed
- 1/4 teaspoon salt
- 6 tablespoons water
- 3 tablespoons chopped fresh parsley
- Toasted sesame seeds for garnish

Let's Get Started:

1. In a food processor, blend the tahini with lemon juice, olive oil, garlic and salt until smooth and creamy.
2. While the machine is running, slowly stream in water until you get a perfectly dip-able consistency.
3. Transfer to a serving bowl and fold in some chopped fresh parsley.
4. Garnish with a drizzle of olive oil and toasted sesame seeds.

Nutrition Facts/Serving: Calories: 106 | Fat: 10g | Carbs: 4g | Protein: 3g

Chocolate Cherry Energy Bites

Serves: 20 Energy Bites   **Prep and Cook Time:** 2hours

Ingredients:

- 1 cup dried cherries
- 1 cup rolled oats
- 1/2 cup dark chocolate chips
- 1/2 cup cashew butter or peanut butter
- 1/4 cup honey
- 1/4 teaspoon vanilla extract

Let's Get Cooking:

1. In a big bowl, put together the oats, dried cherries, chocolate chips, cashew butter (or peanut butter), honey, and vanilla extract. Mix and stir really well until everything is combined and it becomes one sticky clump.
2. Put that sticky mixture into the fridge for around 30 minutes. Making it cold will make it easier to shape into little balls later.
3. After 30 minutes in the fridge, take the mixture out. Use your hands or a small scoop to make small ball shapes, about bite-size. If the mixture is too sticky to work with, you can wet your hands a little with water so it doesn't stick as much.
4. Once you've made all the little balls, put them back in the fridge for 20 more minutes. This will help them hold their shape better.
5. After that 20 minutes in the fridge, the energy bites are ready to eat! You can also put them in a sealed container and keep them in the fridge for up to one week. Or you can freeze them to keep for longer.

Nutrition Facts/Serving: Calories: 108 | Carbs: 12g | Protein: 2g | Fat: 6g

Air Fryer Sweet Potato Chips

Serves: 2-4   **Prep and Cook Time:** 18mins

Ingredients:

- 2 medium-sized sweet potatoes
- 1 tablespoon of high-heat oil (avocado oil, olive oil, or coconut oil)
- Salt and pepper to taste
- Seasonings like dried herbs, chili powder, or garlic powder (optional)

Let's Get Cooking:

1. Preheat your air fryer to 350°F (175°C).
2. Wash the sweet potatoes and slice them into very thin rounds, about 1/8 inch thick, using a sharp knife or mandoline slicer.
3. In a large bowl, toss the sweet potato slices with the oil, salt, and pepper until evenly coated. Add any additional seasonings if desired.
4. Place the slices in a single layer in the air fryer basket. You may need to work in batches to avoid overcrowding.
5. Cook for 6-8 minutes, or until the chips start to crisp. Keep an eye on them to prevent burning.
6. Allow the chips to cool on a wire rack to maintain their crispiness.
7. Let me know if you need any other snacks or recipes humanized! Getting that friendly, personal tone can make all the difference.

Nutrition Facts/Serving: Calories: 150 | Fat: 3.5g | Carbs: 23g | Protein: 2g

The Ultimate Avocado Tuna Salad

Serves: 2-3   **Prep Time (No Cooking):** 10mins

Ingredients:

- 1 ripe avocado (about 150 grams)
- 1/4 cup low-fat Greek yogurt (about 60 grams)
- 1 tablespoon lemon juice (about 15 ml)
- 2 tablespoons chopped fresh parsley (about 7.6 grams)
- 1/2 teaspoon garlic powder (about 1.5 grams)
- 1/4 teaspoon paprika (about 0.6 grams)
- Salt and pepper to taste (about 1/4 teaspoon each)
- 1 can of tuna in water (drained, about 140 grams)
- 1/4 cup diced onion or celery (about 40 grams)

Let's Get Started:

1. In a bowl, use a fork or masher to squash up the avocado really well until it's all mashed.

2. Add in the Greek yogurt and mix it together with the mashed avocado until it becomes one smooth, creamy mixture.

3. Put in the lemon juice, parsley, garlic powder, paprika, salt, and pepper. Stir and mix everything together so all the flavors are combined.

4. Carefully fold in the tuna and the diced onion or celery pieces. Gently mix them in without mashing up the tuna too much.

Nutrition Facts/Serving: Calories: 220 | Protein: 20g | Fat: 12g | Carbs: 9g

Vegan Chocolate Banana Bites

Serves: 24 Banana Bites   **Prep and Cook Time:** 2hours 30mins

Ingredients:

- 3 large bananas
- 1/4 cup natural peanut butter (chunky or smooth)
- 3/4 cup vegan chocolate chips

Let's Get Cooking:

1. Peel the banana skins off the bananas. Cut each banana into two long halves.
2. Take some peanut butter and spread it on each banana half.
3. Put the two peanut butter covered banana halves together to make a "sandwich".
4. Cut each banana "sandwich" into 8 round slices.
5. Put all the banana slice bites onto a tray or baking sheet lined with parchment or wax paper. Put this in the freezer for at least 2 hours or overnight.
6. Put the chocolate chips into a bowl that is safe for the microwave. Melt the chips in the microwave by heating in 15 second intervals, stopping to stir each time, until fully melted (around 1 to 1.5 minutes total).
7. Take the frozen banana bites and dip half of each one into the melted chocolate.
8. Let the chocolate covered part sit until the chocolate is firm and hardened. If not eating right away, put them back in the freezer.

Nutrition Facts/Serving: Calories: 58 | Fat: 3g | Carbs: 8g | Protein: 1g

Fruit & Nut Energy Balls

Serves: 20 Energy Balls   **Prep Time (No Cooking):** 15mins

Ingredients:

- 1 cup mixed nuts (such as almonds, walnuts, and cashews)
- 1 cup mixed dried fruits (such as figs, apricots, and dates)
- 1/4 cup seeds (such as sunflower or pumpkin seeds)
- 2 tablespoons honey or maple syrup (for vegan option)
- 1 teaspoon vanilla extract
- A pinch of salt

Let's Get Cooking:

1. Put the nuts and seeds in a food processor. Chop them up until they are in really small pieces.
2. Add the dried fruits, honey (or maple syrup if using that), vanilla extract, and a little salt to the food processor with the chopped nuts/seeds.
3. Chop it again until everything is well combined into one sticky mixture when you press on it.
4. Take small portions of the sticky mixture and roll them into little ball shapes, about 1 inch across.
5. Put all the little balls onto a baking sheet lined with parchment paper. Put the baking sheet into the fridge for at least 30 minutes so the balls can firm up and hold their shape.

Nutrition Facts/Serving: Calories: 120 | Protein: 3g | Fat: 8g | Carbs: 12g

Vibrant Roasted Beet Hummus

Serves: 10   **Prep Time (No Cooking):** 10mins

Ingredients:

- 1 (15 ounce) can no-salt-added chickpeas, rinsed (425g)
- 8 ounces roasted beets, coarsely chopped and patted dry (227g)
- 1/4 cup tahini (60ml)
- 1/4 cup extra-virgin olive oil (60ml)
- 1/4 cup lemon juice (60ml)
- 1 clove garlic
- 1 teaspoon ground cumin (2.6g)
- 1/2 teaspoon salt (2.5g)

Let's Get Cooking:

1. Put chickpeas, beets, tahini, oil, lemon juice, garlic, cumin, and salt into a food processor bowl.
2. Turn on the food processor and blend everything together until it becomes one very smooth mixture. This will probably take around 2 to 3 minutes of blending.
3. Scoop the smooth hummus into a bowl. You can eat it with veggie sticks, pita chips, or raw veggie pieces for dipping.

Nutrition Facts/Serving: Calories: 133 | Fat: 10g | Carbs: 10g | Protein: 3g

No-Bake Banana Oat Bites

Serves: 16 Bites   **Prep Time (No Cooking):** 15mins

Ingredients:

- 2 ripe bananas
- 2 cups rolled oats (gluten-free if required)
- 1/4 cup almond butter
- 1/4 cup maple syrup
- 2 tablespoons raw cacao nibs
- 1/2 teaspoon ground cinnamon

Let's Get Started:

1. Peel the banana skins off and put the bananas in a medium bowl. Use a fork to mash up the bananas really well until smooth.
2. Put all the other ingredients into the bowl with the mashed bananas. Use a spoon or flat utensil to mix and stir everything together until fully combined.
3. Use a teaspoon to scoop up small portions of the mixed dough. Roll each portion between your hands to shape it into little balls, about 1 1/2 inches across.
4. Put all the little dough balls onto a tray lined with parchment paper. Put the tray into the fridge for 2 hours so the balls can firm up.

Nutrition Facts/Serving: Calories: 94 | Fat: 3g | Carbs: 15g | Protein: 2g

The Ultimate Homemade Trail Mix

Serves: 4 Cups

Ingredients:

- 1/2 cup almonds
- 1/2 cup pecans
- 1/2 cup cashews
- 1/2 cup peanuts
- 1/4 cup coconut flakes
- 1/4 cup raisins
- 1/4 cup M&M's or dark chocolate chips (for a healthier option)

Let's Get Cooking:

1. In a large bowl, combine the nuts, coconut flakes, and raisins.
2. Stir the mixture until well combined.
3. Add the M&M's or dark chocolate chips and mix again.
4. Transfer the trail mix to an airtight container or jar and store at room temperature.

Nutrition Facts/Serving: Calories: 150 | Protein: 4g | Fat: 12g | Carbs: 9g

DESSERT AND SWEET TREATS

Yogurt with Fresh Strawberries and Honey

Serves: 1   **Prep Time (no cooking):** 5mins

Ingredients:

- 1 cup non-fat plain Greek yogurt

- ½ cup fresh strawberries, sliced

- 1 tablespoon honey (preferably raw)

Let's Get Cooking:

1. Wash the strawberries under cool water, then remove the stems and slice them.

2. In a serving bowl, scoop 1 cup of non-fat plain Greek yogurt.

3. Arrange the sliced strawberries on top of the yogurt.

4. Drizzle with Honey: Drizzle 1 tablespoon of honey over the strawberries and yogurt.

5. Serve Immediately: Enjoy your dish fresh for the best flavor and texture.

Nutrition Facts/Serving: Calories: 150 | Fat: 2g | Carbs: 26g | Protein: 8g

2. Light Pumpkin Pie

Serves: 8   **Prep and Cook Time:** 1hour 15mins

Ingredients:

- 1 can of pumpkin puree (15 oz)
- 1 can of low-fat evaporated milk (12 oz)
- 2 large eggs
- ½ cup packed brown sugar
- 2 teaspoons pumpkin pie spice (or mix ground cinnamon, nutmeg, ginger, and cloves)
- 1 teaspoon vanilla extract
- ½ teaspoon salt
- 1 pre-made whole wheat pie crust (9-inch)

Let's Get Cooking:

1. Heat up your oven to 425°F (220°C).
2. Put the pumpkin puree, evaporated milk, and eggs into a big bowl. Beat them together until smooth and blended. Add the brown sugar, pumpkin pie spice, vanilla extract, and salt to the pumpkin mixture. Stir it all together really well so everything is fully mixed in.
3. If using a frozen pre-made whole wheat pie crust, take it out of the freezer and let it thaw for 10-15 minutes until it's soft. Put the pie crust onto a baking sheet so it's easy to move in and out of the oven.
4. Scoop the pumpkin filling into the pie crust and use a spatula to smooth out the top.
5. First, bake it at 425°F for 15 minutes. Then, turn the oven down to 350°F (175°C) and bake for 40 more minutes, or until a knife poked into the middle comes out clean.

6. Let the pie cool off on a wire rack for at least 2 hours so it can set properly. Cut it into 8 slices and serve. If you want, you can add a dollop of low-fat whipped cream or Greek yogurt on top.

Nutrition Facts/Serving: Calories: 180 | Protein: 6g | Fat: 5g | Carbs: 28g

Tahini and Almond Cookies

Serves: 12 cookies   **Prep and Cook Time:** 25mins

Ingredients:

- 1 cup almond flour
- 1/2 cup tahini (sesame seed paste)
- 1/4 cup honey or maple syrup (for a less sweet version, reduce to 3 tablespoons)
- 1 teaspoon vanilla extract
- 1/4 teaspoon salt
- 1/2 teaspoon baking soda
- 1/4 cup sliced almonds (Optional)

Let's Get Cooking:

1. Preheat your oven to 350°F (175°C). Place parchment paper on a baking sheet to avoid sticking.
2. In a small bowl, combine the almond flour, salt, and baking soda. Stir these together until evenly mixed.
3. In a larger mixing bowl, blend the tahini, honey (or maple syrup), and vanilla extract. Whisk these together until you get a smooth, consistent mixture.
4. Gradually add the dry ingredients to the wet ingredients, stirring continuously until a cohesive dough forms.

5. Use a tablespoon to scoop portions of the dough, then roll them into balls. Place these on the prepared baking sheet, spaced about 2 inches apart.

6. Gently press each ball with the back of a fork to slightly flatten and create a crosshatch pattern. If using, sprinkle the tops with sliced almonds.

7. Bake in the preheated oven for about 10 minutes, or until the edges are golden and the centers are set.

8. Once those cookies are out of the oven, don't rush them off the baking sheet just yet! Let them have a little rest period on the hot sheet for about 5 minutes. This allows them to firm up slightly before you transfer them. After that short rest, carefully move the cookies over to a wire cooling rack.

Nutrition Facts/Serving: Calories: 160 | Protein: 4g | Fat: 11g | Carbs: 13g

Fruit Skewers with Cheesecake Yogurt Dip

Servings: 12 skewers   **Prep Time (no cooking):** 15mins

Ingredients:

For the Skewers:

- 1 pint strawberries, washed and hulled
- 1 pint blueberries, washed
- 2 large bananas, peeled and sliced into coins
- 12 wooden skewers

For the Cheesecake Yogurt Dip:

- 1 cup plain low-fat Greek yogurt
- 2 tablespoons honey
- 1 teaspoon pure vanilla extract
- 1 tablespoon lemon juice
- 2 tablespoons low-fat cream cheese, softened

Let's Get Cooking:

1. If the strawberries are very big, cut them into halves so they are bite-size pieces. Slice the bananas into thick round slices so they don't break when putting them on the skewers. Leave the blueberries whole.

2. Start making the skewers by putting a strawberry half on first, then a banana slice, then a few blueberries. Keep going in that pattern until the skewer is full, leaving a little space at the bottom to hold onto. Arrange the fruit in a red, white, and blue pattern to look like the American flag colors.

3. In a medium bowl, mix together the Greek yogurt, honey, vanilla extract, lemon juice, and softened cream cheese. Whisk it all together until it becomes one smooth, creamy mixture.

4. Put the fruit skewers and the dip in the fridge until ready to eat. This keeps the fruit fresh and the dip thick. When ready, take them out and you can eat the fruit skewers by dipping them in the creamy yogurt dip.

Nutrition Facts/Serving: Calories: 70 | Protein: 2g | Fat: 1g | Carbs: 14g

Pear-Cranberry Pie with Oatmeal Streusel

Servings: 8   **Prep and Cook Time:** 1hour 15mins

Ingredients:

For Filling:

- 4 medium pears (peeled and sliced)
- 1 cup fresh cranberries
- ¼ cup granulated sugar
- 2 tablespoons whole wheat flour
- 1 teaspoon ground cinnamon
- ½ teaspoon ground nutmeg
- 1 pre-made whole wheat pie crust (9-inch)

For Oatmeal Streusel Topping:

- ½ cup rolled oats
- ¼ cup whole wheat flour
- ¼ cup packed brown sugar
- ¼ cup unsalted butter, chilled and cut into small pieces
- ½ teaspoon ground cinnamon

Let's Get Cooking:

1. Heat up your oven to 375°F (190°C).

2. Mix together the sliced pears, cranberries, white sugar, 2 tablespoons of whole wheat flour, 1 teaspoon cinnamon, and nutmeg in a big bowl until the fruit is evenly coated. Scoop this fruit mixture into the pre-made whole wheat pie crust and spread it out evenly.

3. Mix the oats, 1/4 cup whole wheat flour, brown sugar, and 1/2 teaspoon cinnamon in another bowl. Use a pastry blender or two

forks to cut in the chilled unsalted butter until the mixture looks like coarse crumbs.

4. Sprinkle this oatmeal crumb topping evenly over the pear-cranberry filling in the pie crust. Put the pie onto a baking sheet to catch any spills and bake it in the oven for about 45 minutes, until the topping is golden brown and the filling is bubbling.

5. Let the pie cool off on a wire rack for at least 30 minutes so it can set before cutting into slices. Serve it warm.

Nutrition Facts/Serving: Calories: 220 | Protein: 3g | Fat: 6g | Carbs: 42g

Oatmeal Walnut Chocolate Chip Cookies

Serves: 24 cookies   **Prep and Cook Time:** 25mins

Ingredients:

- 1 cup whole wheat flour
- 1½ cups rolled oats
- ½ teaspoon baking soda
- ¼ teaspoon salt
- ½ cup unsalted butter, softened
- ½ cup brown sugar
- ¼ cup granulated sugar
- 1 large egg1 teaspoon vanilla extract
- ½ cup walnuts, chopped
- ½ cup dark chocolate chips

Let's Get Cooking

1. Get that oven hot at 350°F. While it's heating, put down some baking paper on a couple of trays. This will make taking the cookies off and cleaning up much easier later!

2. Mix together the whole wheat flour, oats, baking soda, and salt in a medium bowl with a whisk or spoon.

3. In a big separate bowl, mix the softened butter with the brown and white sugars using a hand mixer. Beat it until it looks light, fluffy, and well-blended this should take around 2-3 minutes.

4. Next, crack in the egg and vanilla extract. Beat again until fully mixed.

5. You can now slowly add in the dry ingredients to the wet ones. Use a rubber spatula to gently mix and fold everything together until just combined. Don't overmix!

6. Add in the crunchy chopped walnuts and chocolate chips for melty pockets of deliciousness. I always sneak in a few extra chocolate chips too.

7. Now use a spoon or cookie scoop to make tablespoon-sized balls of dough onto the prepared baking trays. If you want flatter cookies, gently press down on them a little with the back of the spoon.

8. Put them in the oven for around 10 minutes. The edges should be lightly browned when they're ready. The middles may still look a tiny bit underbaked, but that's perfect!

9. As soon as the cookies come out, leave them right on the hot baking tray for 5 minutes. This lets them keep baking and firming up a little before you move them.

10. Once those 5 minutes are up, use a spatula to move the cookies onto a wire rack. Let them fully cool down before eating! This helps give that perfect, delicious cookie texture.

Nutrition Facts/Cookie: Calories: 115 | Protein: 2g | Fat: 5g | Carbs: 16g

Milk Chocolate Pudding

Servings: 4   **Prep and Cook Time:** 2hrs 20mins

Ingredients

- 2 cups low-fat milk (1% milk fat)
- 2 tablespoons cornstarch
- ⅓ cup cocoa powder (unsweetened)
- ¼ cup honey (or you can use an alternative like maple syrup to taste)
- ½ teaspoon vanilla extract
- A pinch of salt

Let's Get Mixing:

1. In a medium pot, make a smooth paste by mixing the cornstarch, cocoa powder, salt, and slowly stirring in about 1/4 cup of milk. Then, slowly pour in the rest of the milk while whisking the whole time to keep the mixture smooth.
2. Put the pot on medium heat. Cook the mixture, stirring it the whole time, until it starts to get thicker and just starts to bubble. This should take around 5-7 minutes. Then, turn the heat down low and keep stirring for two more minutes.
3. Take the pot off the heat. Mix in the honey and vanilla extract until everything is combined well.
4. Spoon the pudding evenly into four separate little bowls or cups. Cover each one with plastic wrap, putting the wrap right on top of the pudding so no hard skin forms. Put them in the fridge for at least 2 hours, or until the pudding is firm and really cold.
5. Once cooled down, you can eat the pudding plain or make it look fancy with grated chocolate, some berries, or a little powdered sugar sprinkled on top.

Nutrition Facts/Serving: Calories: 150 | Protein: 5g | Fat: 3g | Carbs: 24g

Lactose-Free Chocolate Pudding

Servings: 4   **Prep and Chill Time:** 2hrs 20mins

Ingredients

- 2 cups lactose-free milk (preferably low-fat or skim)
- 3 tablespoons unsweetened cocoa powder
- 2 tablespoons cornstarch
- ¼ cup maple syrup (you can also use honey or any sugar substitute)
- 1 teaspoon vanilla extract
- Pinch of salt

Let's Get Mixing:

1. In a medium pot, mix together the cocoa powder, cornstarch, and a little bit of salt. Stir these dry ingredients together so there are no lumps.
2. Then, slowly pour in the milk that doesn't have lactose (milk sugar), while stirring the whole time. This will keep the mixture smooth without any lumps.
3. Put the pot on medium heat and keep stirring the mixture as it cooks. As it heats up, add in the maple syrup and keep on stirring. The mixture will slowly get thicker this should take around 5-10 minutes. Once it has the thickness of a thick sauce, take it off the heat.
4. After taking the pot off the heat, stir in the vanilla extract. This will add great flavor without cooking off the vanilla taste.
5. Spoon the pudding into four separate little bowls or one big bowl. Cover with plastic wrap, pressing the wrap right onto the top of the pudding so no hard skin forms. Put it in the fridge for at least 2 hours, until the pudding is firm and cold.
6. Serve the chocolate pudding when it's nice and chilled. If you want, you can make it look fancy by adding some fresh raspberries or

sprinkling grated dark chocolate on top for extra flavor and decoration.

Nutrition Facts/Serving: Calories: 140 | Protein: 5g | Fat: 4g | Carbs: 24g

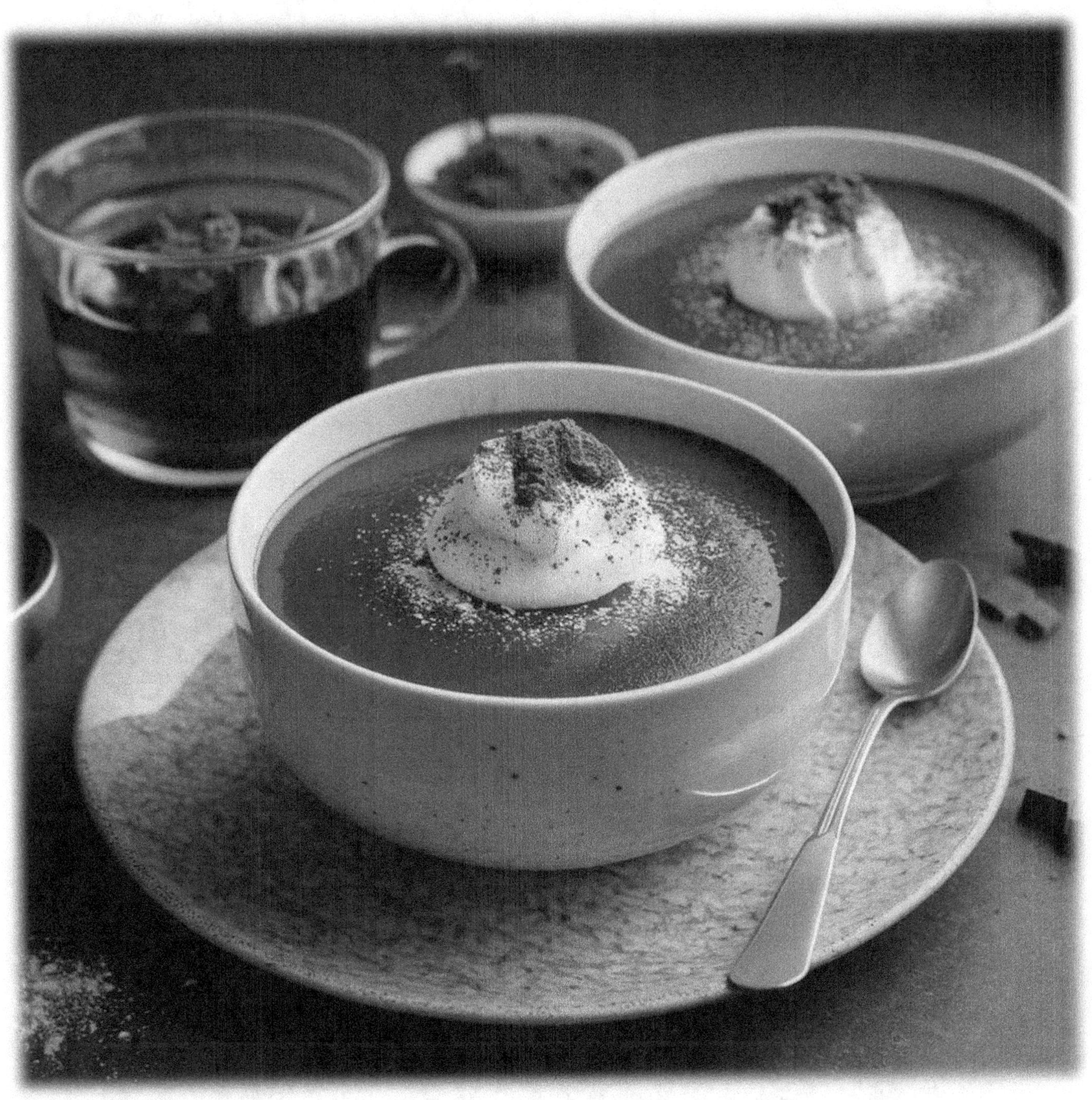

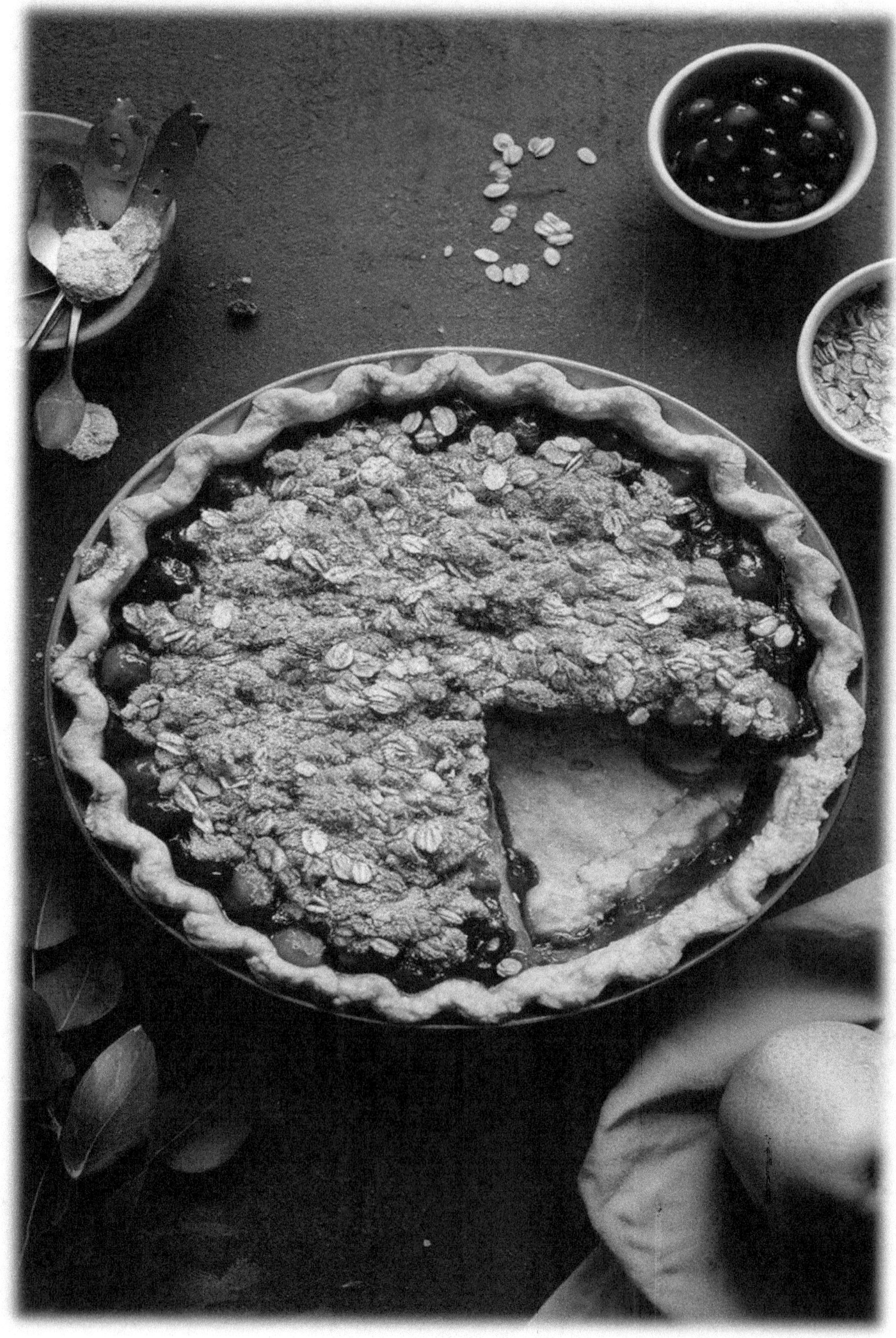

CONCLUSION

Reflecting on the Journey of Health and Well-being

Adopting the DASH Diet is more than changing what you eat; it's about transforming how you think about food and its impact on your body and mind. Throughout this book, we've explored the key components of the DASH Diet, from stocking your kitchen to preparing meals that not only nourish but also delight. This journey has been about laying a foundation for a lifestyle that promotes sustained health and vitality.

Reaffirming the Benefits of the DASH Diet

As we reflect on what we've learned, it's important to remember why the DASH Diet is so beneficial:

✓ The diet's low sodium, high potassium, and balanced nutrient intake significantly reduce hypertension and improve heart health.

✓ Beyond heart health, the DASH Diet supports weight management, reduces cancer risk, improves bone health, and stabilizes blood sugar levels, contributing to overall improved health.

✓ By improving physical health, the DASH Diet also supports mental and emotional well-being, enhancing mood and energy levels.

The end of this book is just the beginning of your ongoing journey with the DASH Diet. Health and dietary needs evolve over time, and staying informed and adaptable is key:

➢ Continue to try new recipes and tweak old favorites to fit the DASH Diet better. Each recipe is a building block in a varied and exciting diet.

➤ Keep up with the latest nutrition research and recommendations to refine your diet further and adjust to new health information as it becomes available.

➤ Join forums, attend workshops, or participate in community groups focused on healthy living to share experiences, recipes, and support

➤ Focus on the quality of the foods you eat, where they come from, and how they benefit your body. Mindful eating practices can enhance your enjoyment and appreciation of food.

➤ Life's unpredictability requires flexibility in your diet. Learning how to make smart food choices in different situations ensure that you can stick to the DASH principles no matter the circumstances.

➤ Build a support system of family, friends, and healthcare providers who understand and support your dietary choices. This network can provide encouragement and motivation.

Final Words of Encouragement

As you continue with the DASH Diet, remember that each day is a new opportunity to nourish your body and mind. Be patient and persistent, and take pride in the positive changes you're making. Your journey to better health is a personal one, and this book aims to be a companion along the way, offering guidance, recipes, and encouragement.

Your Thoughts Matter

I hope you have found good foods and comfort in the recipes and guidance offered in this cookbook. My goal was to provide you recipes that serve as a source of support and strength on your journey to feeling well.

If you have a moment, I would be very thankful if you could share your thoughts about this cookbook. Your feedback is very valuable, not only to me but to others who may find peace in these pages. Whether it is a certain recipe that became your new favorite or any suggestions for how this cookbook can be better, I am eager to hear from you.

Please consider leaving a review on Amazon or share your thoughts and experiences on any social media platform of your choice. Your voice has the power to inspire and assist others who are finding their own paths.

Here is to many more shared meals and moments of hope and healing.

Cheers...

Cynthia Ashcroft
Author

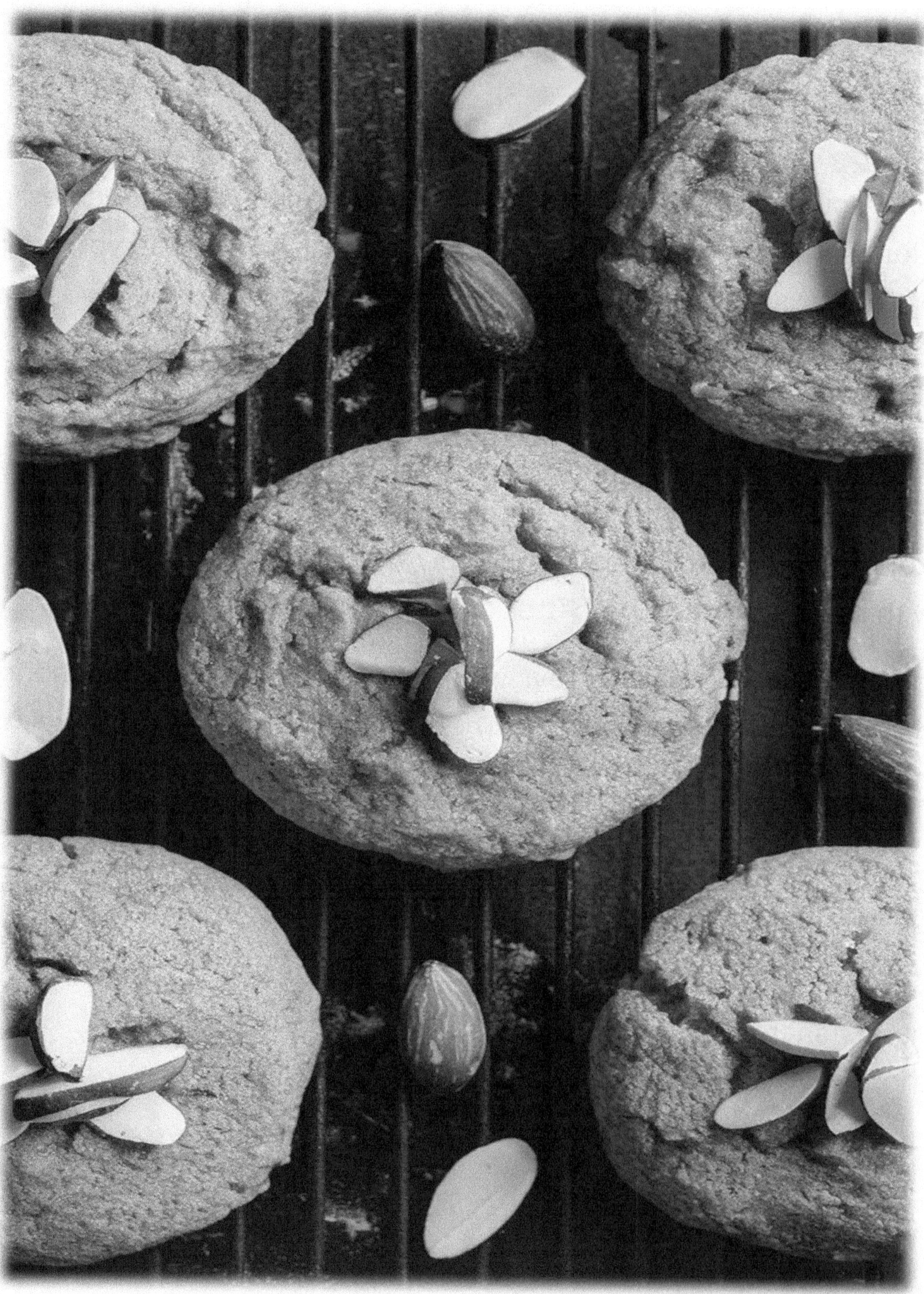

30 DAYS DASH DIET MEAL PLAN

Day 1

Breakfast: Peanut Butter Overnight Oats

Lunch: Chipotle-Lime Cauliflower Taco Bowls

Dinner: Chickpea Pasta with Mushrooms & Kale

Snack: Chewy, Nutty Apricot Granola Bars

Day 2

Breakfast: Muesli Scones

Lunch: Veggie & Hummus Sandwich

Dinner: Sheet-Pan Chili-Lime Salmon with Potatoes & Peppers

Snack: Classic Greek Tahini Dip

Day 3

Breakfast: Healthy Breakfast Cookies

Lunch: Spinach & Strawberry Meal-Prep Salad

Dinner: Pork Paprikash with Cauliflower Rice

Snack: Chocolate Cherry Energy Bites

Day 4

Breakfast: Mushroom Spinach Omelet

Lunch: Smoked Salmon Salad Nicoise

Dinner: One-Pot Garlicky Shrimp & Spinach

Snack: Air Fryer Sweet Potato Chips

Day 5

Breakfast: Blueberry Banana Spelt Muffins

Lunch: Sweet Potato, Kale & Chicken Salad with Peanut Dressing

Dinner: Beef & Bean Sloppy Joes

Snack: The Ultimate Avocado Tuna Salad

Day 6

Breakfast: 5-Ingredient Buckwheat Crepes

Lunch: Meal-Prep Vegan Lettuce Wraps

Dinner: Seared Scallops with White Bean Ragu & Charred Lemon

Snack: Vegan Chocolate Banana Bites

Day 7

Breakfast: Blueberry Yogurt Multigrain Pancakes

Lunch: Mason Jar Power Salad with Chickpeas & Tuna

Dinner: Nutrient-Packed Quinoa Power Bowl

Snack: Fruit & Nut Energy Balls

Day 8

Breakfast: Sweet Potato Oat Waffles

Lunch: Winter Kale & Quinoa Salad with Avocado

Dinner: Summer Veggie & Egg Scramble

Snack: Vibrant Roasted Beet Hummus

Day 9

Breakfast: Sweet Potato and Black Bean Breakfast Burrito

Lunch: Vegan Superfood Grain Bowls

Dinner: Chipotle Chicken Quinoa Burrito Bowls

Snack: No-Bake Banana Oat Bites

Day 10

Breakfast: Ezekiel Bread French Toast

Lunch: Tomato, Cucumber & White-Bean Salad with Basil Vinaigrette

Dinner: Sizzling Beef & Baby Bok Choy Stir-Fry

Snack: The Ultimate Homemade Trail Mix

Day 11

Breakfast: Vegetable Hash with Poached Eggs

Lunch: Chimichurri Noodle Bowls

Dinner: Pan-Seared Steak with Crispy Herb Salad

Snack: Yogurt with Fresh Strawberries and Honey

Day 12

Breakfast: Open Face Breakfast Sandwich

Lunch: White Bean & Veggie Salad

Dinner: Power Up with this Nutrient-Packed Chopped Salad

Snack: Light Pumpkin Pie

Day 13

Breakfast: Turkey Bacon and Egg Breakfast Tacos

Lunch: Lemon-Roasted Vegetable Hummus Bowls

Dinner: Chickpea Pasta with Mushrooms & Kale

Snack: Tahini and Almond Cookies

Day 14

Breakfast: Smoked Salmon on Whole Grain Toast

Lunch: Mixed Greens with Lentils & Sliced Apple

Dinner: Sheet-Pan Chili-Lime Salmon with Potatoes & Peppers

Snack: Fruit Skewers with Cheesecake Yogurt Dip

Day 15

Breakfast: Southwest Tofu Scramble

Lunch: Rainbow Grain Bowl with Cashew Tahini Sauce

Dinner: Pork Paprikash with Cauliflower Rice

Snack: Pear-Cranberry Pie with Oatmeal Streusel

Day 16

Breakfast: Peanut Butter Overnight Oats

Lunch: Chipotle-Lime Cauliflower Taco Bowls

Dinner: One-Pot Garlicky Shrimp & Spinach

Snack: Oatmeal Walnut Chocolate Chip Cookies

Day 17

Breakfast: Muesli Scones

Lunch: Veggie & Hummus Sandwich

Dinner: Beef & Bean Sloppy Joes

Snack: Milk Chocolate Pudding

Day 18

Breakfast: Healthy Breakfast Cookies

Lunch: Spinach & Strawberry Meal-Prep Salad

Dinner: Seared Scallops with White Bean Ragu & Charred Lemon

Snack: Lactose-Free Chocolate Pudding

Day 19

Breakfast: Mushroom Spinach Omelet

Lunch: Smoked Salmon Salad Nicoise

Dinner: Power Up with this Nutrient-Packed Chopped Salad

Snack: Chewy, Nutty Apricot Granola Bars

Day 20

Breakfast: Blueberry Banana Spelt Muffins

Lunch: Sweet Potato, Kale & Chicken Salad with Peanut Dressing

Dinner: Nutrient-Packed Quinoa Power Bowl

Snack: Classic Greek Tahini Dip

Day 21

Breakfast: 5-Ingredient Buckwheat Crepes

Lunch: Meal-Prep Vegan Lettuce Wraps

Dinner: Summer Veggie & Egg Scramble

Snack: Chocolate Cherry Energy Bites

Day 22

Breakfast: Blueberry Yogurt Multigrain Pancakes

Lunch: Mason Jar Power Salad with Chickpeas & Tuna

Dinner: Chipotle Chicken Quinoa Burrito Bowls

Snack: Air Fryer Sweet Potato Chips

Day 23

Breakfast: Sweet Potato Oat Waffles

Lunch: Winter Kale & Quinoa Salad with Avocado

Dinner: Sizzling Beef & Baby Bok Choy Stir-Fry

Snack: The Ultimate Avocado Tuna Salad

Day 24

Breakfast: Sweet Potato and Black Bean Breakfast Burrito

Lunch: Vegan Superfood Grain Bowls

Dinner: Pan-Seared Steak with Crispy Herb Salad

Snack: Vegan Chocolate Banana Bites

Day 25:

Breakfast: Ezekiel Bread French Toast

Lunch: Tomato, Cucumber & White-Bean Salad with Basil Vinaigrette

Dinner: Chickpea Pasta with Mushrooms & Kale

Snack: Fruit & Nut Energy Balls

Day 26:

Breakfast: Vegetable Hash with Poached Eggs

Lunch: Chimichurri Noodle Bowls

Dinner: Sheet-Pan Chili-Lime Salmon with Potatoes & Peppers

Snack: Vibrant Roasted Beet Hummus

Day 27:

Breakfast: Open Face Breakfast Sandwich

Lunch: White Bean & Veggie Salad

Dinner: Pork Paprikash with Cauliflower Rice

Snack: No-Bake Banana Oat Bites

Day 28:

Breakfast: Turkey Bacon and Egg Breakfast Tacos

Lunch: Lemon-Roasted Vegetable Hummus Bowls

Dinner: One-Pot Garlicky Shrimp & Spinach

Snack: The Ultimate Homemade Trail Mix

Day 29:

Breakfast: Smoked Salmon on Whole Grain Toast

Lunch: Mixed Greens with Lentils & Sliced Apple

Dinner: Beef & Bean Sloppy Joes

Snack: Yogurt with Fresh Strawberries and Honey

Day 30:

Breakfast: Southwest Tofu Scramble

Lunch: Rainbow Grain Bowl with Cashew Tahini Sauce

Dinner: Seared Scallops with White Bean Ragu & Charred Lemon

Snack: Light Pumpkin Pie

MONDAY	TUESDAY
WEDNESDAY	THURSDAY
FRIDAY	SATURDAY
SUNDAY	*notes*

MONDAY	TUESDAY
WEDNESDAY	THURSDAY
FRIDAY	SATURDAY
SUNDAY	*notes*

<table>
<tr><td>MONDAY</td><td>TUESDAY</td></tr>
<tr><td>WEDNESDAY</td><td>THURSDAY</td></tr>
<tr><td>FRIDAY</td><td>SATURDAY</td></tr>
<tr><td>SUNDAY</td><td>*notes*</td></tr>
</table>

MONDAY

TUESDAY

WEDNESDAY

THURSDAY

FRIDAY

SATURDAY

SUNDAY

notes